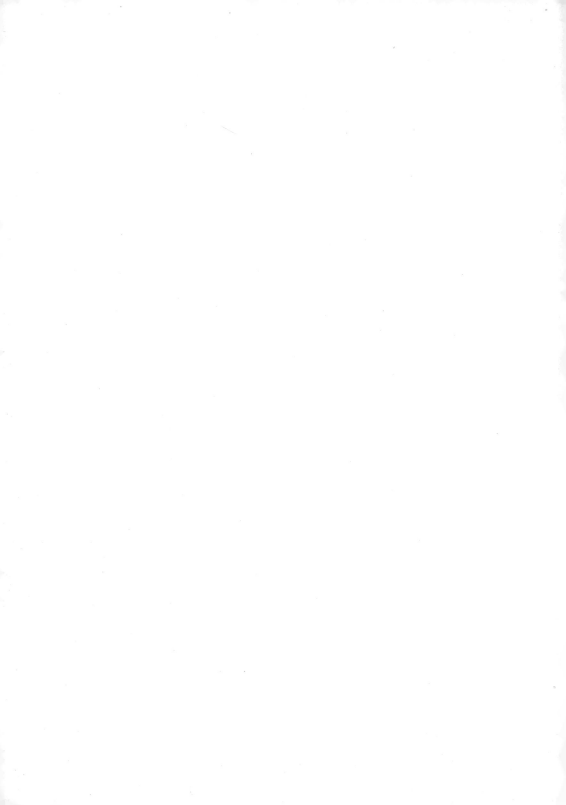

Lita Linzer Schwartz, PhD
Florence W. Kaslow, PhD
Editors

Welcome Home!
An International and Nontraditional Adoption Reader

Pre-publication
REVIEWS,
COMMENTARIES,
EVALUATIONS . . .

"**S**chwartz and Kaslow have captured both the heart and mind of international and nontraditional adoption. They raise questions one would never think to ask and carefully guide readers through the answers. Not only is this text filled with essential information, it also appeals to the heart. It's filled with touching, personal, first-person narratives about the good news, the bad news, and the real news of adoption. 'Coming Home from China,' by Margaret Moro, for example, is a detailed description of the process of adopting a child. She takes us from the decision to adopt a Chinese baby and her struggle with social justice issues through seemingly never-ending paperwork, disappointments, and finally the trip to China to meet her beautiful young daughter. This story is both touching and informative. Anyone considering international or nontraditional adoption or who has already adopted should read this book. It gives new insights into what it really means to be a family, and what a combination of love and commitment can do to change lives."

Daniel Gottlieb, PhD
Family Therapist;
Columnist, *Philadelphia Inquirer;*
Author, *Voices in the Family*
and *Voices of Conflict, Voices of Healing*

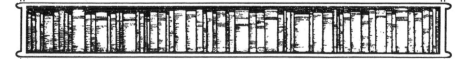

More pre-publication
REVIEWS, COMMENTARIES, EVALUATIONS . . .

"*Welcome Home!*, edited by Dr. Lita Schwartz and Dr. Florence Kaslow, is an interesting and unique addition to adoption literature. By allowing the voices of adoptive parents, grandparents, and siblings to be heard, the book gives valuable, but all-too-infrequently considered, firsthand accounts of the challenges and rewards of international and nontraditional adoption. Above and beyond the requisite practical information the book provides, the heartfelt insights and analyses that the adoptive parents offer about their decision-making processes and their ongoing lives as adoptive families are invaluable to new and prospective parents. This book should be required reading for anyone contemplating an international or nontraditional adoption."

Shelley Kapnek Rosenberg, EdD
Author, *Adoption and the Jewish Family: Contemporary Perspectives*

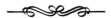

"*A* welcome addition to the annals of literature devoted to the subject of adoption, *Welcome Home!* is unique in that it chronicles the cases of children adopted from outside of the United States—from their parents' point of view. In addition, the book authoritatively presents and clearly describes the hurdles encountered in such international adoptions. More than any other text I have read on the topic, *Welcome Home!* argues quite incisively and, in a simple style, illustrates the key dilemmas faced by these new families—among them the need to overcome social barriers while at the same time retaining many of the cultural differences between the adopted country and the child's original home. Such matters are at the core of the book.

The editors are to be commended for their judicious selection of subjects and case studies, conveying testimonials of both satisfaction and bureaucratic frustrations that accompany the often-protracted international adoption process. As a physician and Voice of America broadcaster to the former Soviet Union, I am often consulted by American couples interested in the prospect of adopting children from that part of the world. To those in search of guidance, I will enthusiastically recommend *Welcome Home!* as required reading before embarking on this quest."

Irene Kelner, MD, PhD
International Broadcaster/Editor,
Voice of America

The Haworth Clinical Practice Press
An Imprint of The Haworth Press, Inc.
New York • London • Oxford

Welcome Home!
An International and Nontraditional Adoption Reader

HAWORTH Marriage and the Family
Terry S. Trepper, PhD
Executive Editor

Welcome Home!
An International and Nontraditional Adoption Reader

Lita Linzer Schwartz, PhD
Florence W. Kaslow, PhD
Editors

The Haworth Clinical Practice Press
An Imprint of The Haworth Press, Inc.
New York • London • Oxford

Published by

The Haworth Clinical Practice Press, an imprint of The Haworth Press, Inc., 10 Alice Street, Binghamton, NY 13904-1580.

Client identities and circumstances have been changed to protect confidentiality.

Cover design by Jennifer M. Gaska.

Cover photo (on left) is of Marianne Cederblad with her children and grandchildren.

Library of Congress Cataloging-in-Publication Data

Welcome home! : an international and nontraditional adoption reader / Lita Linzer Schwartz, Florence Kaslow, Editors.
    p.   cm.
Includes bibliographical references and index.
    ISBN 0-7890-1773-3 (cloth : alk. paper)—ISBN 0-7890-1774-1 (pbk. : alk. paper)
    1. Adoption—United States. 2. Intercountry adoption—United States. I. Schwartz, Lita Linzer.
II. Kaslow, Florence Whiteman.
    HV875.55.W465 2004
    362.73'4'0973—dc21
                                                                    2003012414

CONTENTS

ABOUT THE EDITORS

Lita Linzer Schwartz, PhD, and **Florence W. Kaslow, PhD,** are co-authors of *The Dynamics of Divorce and Painful Partings.* Between them, they have authored or edited 40 books and numerous book chapters and scholarly articles.

Dr. Schwartz is Distinguished Professor Emerita from Penn State, where she taught at Abington (formerly the Penn State Ogontz campus). She holds a Diplomate in Forensic Psychology from the American Board of Professional Psychology and is a Fellow of the American Psychological Association.

Dr. Kaslow is director of the Florida Couples and Family Institute, and president of Kaslow Associates in Palm Beach Gardens, Florida. She is also Visiting Professor of Medical Psychology in Psychiatry at Duke University Medical Center and Visiting Professor of Psychology at Florida Institute of Technology. In 2000, Dr. Kaslow received the American Psychology Association's Award for Distinguished Contribution to the Advancement of International Psychology. She is board certified in clinical, family, and forensic psychology.

CONTRIBUTORS

Elizabeth Allen, age forty-eight, lives and works in Washington, DC. She leads two lives, one professional as an attorney for the U.S. government specializing in environmental and administrative law and the other highly gratifying, as the single mother of four children, ages ten, eight, seven, and four, each of whom joined the family through adoption. She has written under a pseudonym to protect the privacy of her children.

Anne is a pseudonym used to protect her daughters' privacy. She became a first-time mother at age fifty, her husband a first-time father at age fifty-one. He is an economist; she is a journalist. She chose the name Anne as a pseudonym because it is her middle name and because one day she found a novena to Saint Anne in a little box of prayers her grandmother had. During the novena she prayed for a daughter. Afterward, she reports having felt a deep peace and knowing that one day she would have a little girl. The surprise came in getting two girls plus a wonderful little boy.

Kurinu Burrugur currently attends Santa Monica College as a sophomore studying interior design. She also works as a professional actress and model and has completed commercials for Nike, Chex Cereal, Crystal Lite, and Philip Morris Youth Smoking Program.

Krista Barragar graduated from the University of California at Santa Cruz in 2000 with a bachelor of arts degree in creative writing. She is currently a freelance writer and works for a graphics and product design company.

Reese Barragar graduated from the University of California at Santa Cruz in 2002 with a bachelor of arts degree and is currently working in film production.

Samantha Barragar is a professional actress, makeup artist, and interior designer. She enjoys creative pursuits and hopes, in the near future, to teach Shakespeare to children.

Karen Klein Berman lives in New York with her husband of more than fifteen years, Jeff, who is a mergers and acquisitions lawyer, their teenage son Matthew, and their preteen daughter Zoe. Berman is currently the national chair of Families for Russian and Ukranian Adoption (FRUA), which also includes families from neighboring countries. More information on FRUA can be found at <www. frua.org>.

Marianne Cederblad, MD, PhD, is a former professor of child and adolescent psychology at the Universities of Umea and Lund in Sweden. Her research areas include intercountry adoptions, studies on stress and resilience, and epidemiological studies on behavior and adaptation of children and adolescents in Sudan, Ethiopia, and Thailand. She is a licensed family therapist and trainer and teaches family therapy in Sweden and abroad.

Kirby Deater-Deckard, PhD, is a coprincipal investigator on the Northeast-Northwest Collaborative Adoption Project, and assistant professor at the Center for Developmental and Health Genetics, Pennsylvania State University.

Pamela Diane Dunne, mother of the four Barragar contributors, holds doctorates in clinical psychology and theater and, in one job, combines the two as director of the Drama Therapy Institute of Los Angeles. She is also a professor of Theatre Arts and Dance at California State University, Los Angeles.

Jeffery Flanagan is a research associate in the Department of Psychology, University of Oregon.

Deborah Johnson, married and the mother of four wonderful children, aged twenty-two years down to five, recently decided to fulfill a lifelong dream. In May 2000, she enrolled in college as a full-time student, pursuing a career in education. After putting off college for twenty years, she finally found the time to follow through with her dream of becoming a teacher. She is also heavily involved in her community and holds several volunteer positions.

Lee Jones, Esq. (pseudonym), is a nonpracticing attorney. She practiced law for ten years and gladly abandoned her career to care for her and her partner's two daughters. She has now returned to work part-time in local government.

Jehoshua Kaufman, MA, father of three beautiful children and husband to Gunillas, is a licensed psychologist and pyschotherapist practicing in Lund, Sweden. He is the director of Sodre Re, a private center for occupation rehabilitation in the south of Sweden.

Paul A. Lipton, PhD, is a postdoctoral fellow at the Center for Developmental and Health Genetics, Pennsylvania State University.

Naomi Moessinger and her husband Fred still live in the house in which their children grew up. She enjoys spending time with their children and grandchildren, who are scattered from New Jersey to Wisconsin to Texas, and traveling with Fred.

Margaret V. Moro, PhD, mother of Gianna and spouse of Joel, is a licensed marriage and family therapist. She is grateful for having studied families prior to creating a family and takes great joy in watching her daughter explore possibilities that were not available to her as a child.

Tina Morris, MD (pseudonym), is a child psychiatrist working in private practice and community mental health. She has been with her partner, Lee Jones, for sixteen years, and they reside in a large southeastern city.

William D. Palmer, JD, is currently an appellate judge sitting on the Fifth District Court of Appeal in Daytona Beach, Florida. Prior to being appointed to the bench in 2000, he was engaged in the private practice of law. His practice primarily focused on civil litigation, mediation, arbitration, and adoption law, including service as counsel to the Children's Home Society of Florida, adoption agencies, and adoptive parents.

Mildred Peterson is ninety-four years of age, mother and grandmother of contributors, and an avid reader, and is enjoying her retirement in Malibu, California.

Stephen A. Petrill, PhD, is a coprincipal investigator for the Northeast-Northwest Collaborative Adoption Project, and an assistant professor at the Center for Developmental and Health Genetics, Pennsylvania State University.

Shirley C. White (pseudonym) was an executive director of a YMCA and of a shelter for preschool-age abused and abandoned children.

She became concerned because there were no foster homes for babies with HIV and other serious conditions. At sixty-five years plus, she converted her home into a foster home and subsequently became an adoptive mother for hard-to-place children. She now has five children, ages seven to forty-eight years.

Sanno Zack is a master's student in the Department of Psychology, Pennsylvania State University.

Foreword

Those who make the conscious decision to become parents through adoption are special indeed. They tend to have the purest of motives in that they either recognize within themselves a strong need to nurture a child or cannot turn away from their awareness of the dire circumstances of particular children. Too often, the purer the motives, the more susceptible a person becomes to fraud and abuse by unscrupulous individuals.

Drs. Kaslow and Schwartz are to be commended for their decision to interpret adoption through the direct experiences of adoptive parents, as well as for including a variety of family configurations across American, multicultural, and intercountry situations. Their book well documents the loving, unselfish spirit of those who decide to adopt and also highlights the difficulties encountered along the way.

As a psychologist and former child care administrator, I am pleased with the emphasis on creating and maintaining a stable home where the child is wanted and cared for, as opposed to concerns that the home must necessarily follow a traditional family model or take into consideration discriminatory factors such as the necessity to match by race and culture. As a legislator, I am particularly interested in the regulations and policies that exist or should exist to protect the rights and interests of all involved in adoptions.

It is important for all interested in adopting a child from another country to know that the Intercountry Adoption Act of 2000 is in place to establish uniform standards and procedures for international adoptions. This act is intended to protect the rights and interests of not only adoptive children but also the birth and adoptive parents. It falls under the direct responsibility of the secretary of state and attorney general and is intended to guard against fraud and other such problems. For example, the secretary of state has the responsibility of seeing that adoption agencies or individuals involved in the application procedures of prospective adoptive parents are accredited. Under this law, those wanting to adopt can obtain a list of accredited adoption agencies and approved persons (see Appendix) as well as the names of agencies or persons to avoid. The importance of working with credible agencies and knowledgeable individuals is stressed throughout the book. The authors and editors also stress that in intercountry adoptions, it is important that children be enabled to leave orphanages to go to adoptive parents as quickly as possible.

Another situation described in this book involves the foster child whose foster parent(s) desire a permanent placement through adoption. This type of adoption can be more difficult than intercountry adoptions because it involves the U.S. child welfare system, which emphasizes working toward reunification and family preservation. However, the Adoption and Safe Families Act of 1997 (ASFA) was passed with the explicit goals of protecting children by not returning them to unsafe homes and ensuring that the legal termination of parental rights procedures are accomplished with little delay. The new federal law, which has been called the most sweeping change in federal child welfare law in nearly twenty years, engendered major changes in laws, policies, procedures, and practices at the state level. Child care agencies now try to limit the length of time children spend in foster care and make every effort to move them into stable, permanent living situations as quickly as possible. In addition, the ASFA created adoption-incentive payments and medical assistance in an effort to increase the adoption of foster children. An additional incentive is given for the adoption of foster children with special needs.

In 1999, the General Accounting Office's (GAO) report "Foster Care: States' Early Experiences Implementing the Adoption and Safe Families Act" stated that, by July of that year, all states were to have in place laws that mirrored the federal legislation or were more stringent than federal law. However, the GAO has since indicated that implementation of these new state laws has not been perfect; rather, some states have lagged behind in ensuring timely termination of parental rights and decisions permitting permanent unimpeded adoptions. The Department of Health and Human Services continues to monitor states' compliance with the federal law and offers assistance to states struggling with implementation.

In closing, I hope this book by Drs. Kaslow and Schwartz will inspire those who want the opportunity to experience the joy of child rearing to consider adopting one of the many children who need a permanent, stable, loving home. After reading the different experiences of the adoptive parents in this book, the reader will find it easier to determine which type of adoption best suits his or her circumstances and interests. Even readers not planning to adopt will benefit greatly from making the journey with these adoptive parents. It is impossible not to feel their joy when the waiting is over and their disappointment when the process fails them. Equally compelling is the warmth and admiration felt for those who have chosen this nontraditional path with a courage that can be explained only by their love for children. The power of this love is dramatically changing the landscape of the family patterns in the United States. The editors are to be commended for helping us keep the focus where it should be: on making every effort possible to ensure that children at risk live instead in a safe environment and with individuals who truly want and love them. I also believe legislators, policymakers, and those working in the broad field of adoption will find the information contained herein illuminating and inspiring for their work.

Ted Strickland, PhD
House of Representatives
Washington, DC

Chapter 1

Opening the Door

Lita Linzer Schwartz

Let us first be clear on terminology: international and multicultural adoption are not synonymous. International adoption usually involves adoptive parents in one country and one or more children from one or more other countries. Multicultural adoption can occur within the boundaries of one country, for example, the United States, where a Caucasian or an African-American couple might choose to adopt a biracial child, or one of Native American extraction, or simply one whose racial, religious, or ethnic background is different from their own. A second area of difference is that with postnewborn adoptions, children abroad may have spent months or years in an orphanage, while those in the United States are more likely to have been in foster care. Depending on the circumstances in each individual case, one situation is not necessarily better than the other. A third difference used to be more apparent than it is today: the age of adoptees from this country versus those from abroad. It used to be that children from overseas were older, whereas American adoptees were infants. With changing practices in the United States concerning the length of time that children may stay in foster care, that difference is not as apparent as it was a few years ago; fewer healthy infants appear to be available for adoption in this country.

These differences are critical factors in the choices prospective adoptive parents make. Some couples contemplating adoption already have one or more biological children; others have no children. Those considering adoption may, or may not, be a heterosexual couple. What all of these people have in common, however, is the desire to bring a child into their homes and hearts and to nurture that child through the years to become as healthy and happy an adult as possible.

WHY ADOPT?

The very first question that a couple (or an individual) needs to raise is "Why do we (I) want to adopt a child?" Adoption of children has been practiced for as long as there have been children whose own parents could not rear them and adults who chose to assume the parental role, even in the absence of a biological tie. Adults choose the adoptive parental role for a variety of reasons—most often, perhaps, because they are struggling with infertility or are unable to carry a pregnancy themselves yet want to be parents. Even with all of the alternative reproductive technologies (ARTs) available today, not every couple wants infertility counseling and treatment, not every couple can be helped by these techniques or can afford to pay for them, and not every couple chooses to follow the ART route to parenthood (Schwartz, 1991). That does not even count same-sex couples or individuals who wish to parent a child but who have no spouse or partner. It should be noted, in addition, that some of the ART procedures used to overcome infertility, especially those involving a third party as donor of sperm or ovum, are against religious law in Roman Catholicism, Orthodox Judaism, Islam, and several Protestant denominations (Broyde, 1998; Molock, 1999; Oz, 1995; Povarsky, 1998).

In married couples it is often the husband who is particularly anxious to perpetuate his family's genetic heritage, a throwback to traditional inheritance practices. If he is fertile but his wife either is unable to carry a pregnancy or has a fertility problem, as was the case, for example, with the Sterns, parents of "Baby M" in the controversial surrogacy case of the mid-1980s, he may view artificial insemination of a woman who will serve as "surrogate mother" to be highly desirable (Schwartz, 1987). His wife would then adopt the resulting baby. In the event of a divorce, however, he might seek custody of the child on the grounds that the child is *his,* not his wife's. On the other hand, if *he* is the infertile member of the couple, he may resist artificial insemination of his wife because the resulting child would not resemble him at all and would, as a result, "advertise" his lack of reproductive ability. This acknowledgment, beginning with being tested for infertility problems, is perceived as a threat especially to the *machismo* of Hispanic Americans (Molock, 1999), although other males may feel their masculinity threatened as well. It might be helpful for the couple to seek counseling to deal with the nonphysiological aspects of the situation, both to help them as a couple and to consider their options (Diamond et al., 1999). Adoption with neither husband nor wife having a biological connection to the child may be the mutually satisfactory choice. Indeed, some couples have decided that if they cannot *both* contribute to the creation of a child, then neither will; they will both be adoptive parents.

It is essential, however, that the couple agree that they are prepared to assume the same responsibilities as biological parents, that the child will become an "unconditional member of the family," and that they will see themselves as the child's *real* parents—for their own sake and for that of the child (Salzer, 1999). The perception of being the child's real parents will obviously be more difficult all around, however, if they adopt an older child who has lived with another family for some years, or a child of a different racial background, than with a newborn or an infant.

Couples or individuals may or may not choose to discuss the possibility of adoption with their parents or friends. It is conceivable that those who would become the adoptee's grandparents may be opposed to the idea, creating family dissension. Where possible, this should be worked out before a couple moves to the next step, although the ultimate choice is theirs. Apropos of grandparenthood, one grandmother-to-be, greeting her daughter, the daughter's fiancé, and the six-year-old Russian girl they were adopting, found herself feeling very grandmotherly toward the child—to her own surprise. She said it was amazing "that biology has so little to do with bonding. It's the mental commitment you make to another human being." That, indeed, is what adoption is all about.

Having Decided to Adopt . . .

Having made their choice, the couple has other questions to address, as well as many that they will be asked by adoption agencies or attorneys or on behalf of the child they may seek to adopt. (In practice, the more criteria they have in terms of their prospective child, the longer it may take to find one.) Some questions may appear to be very simple but are critical (as Berman points out in Chapter 10):

- What age child do we want to adopt? Do we want a newborn baby, an infant, a toddler, or an older child? Can we care for a newborn?

- Do we have a preference for a boy or a girl? If so, why?
- Do we want a child who looks like one or both of us?
- Does the child have to come from a particular religious or ethnic background?

Up to this point, the prospective parents are dealing with the kinds of possible adoptees who, in years past, were traditionally available in the United States to those who met adoption agency criteria in terms of age, education, length of marriage, cause of infertility, employment arrangements, income, potential caretaking responsibilities, and other factors. Because of the changes that have occurred in the past few decades with respect to the increase in unmarried mothers, especially young white women, now choosing to raise their children (as many young minority group women have done for years rather than placing them for adoption), even those who satisfy agency requirements might have to wait five years or more until a newborn or an infant is found for them to adopt. That leads to additional issues for them, as well as for those who fail to meet agency criteria:

- Do we want an open adoption?
- Would we consider a special needs child?
- Might we consider a child from another country? Which country or countries?
- Would we consider a biracial child or one of a race different from our own?
- If we are willing to adopt a child who will look nothing like us (i.e., another racial background), what is our motive?
- How will we handle the child's questions about this in later years?

The adoption scene has changed markedly in the United States in the past few decades so that prospective parents need to recognize that among the infants available for adoption, many are the children of substance-addicted mothers or of parents with HIV/AIDS. Is the couple prepared to deal with the possible negative effects of these conditions on the child? Many thousands of children in foster care are only now being released for adoption, in recognition of the fact that they will never be returned to their biological parents because of persistent problems in these homes. These children may have been well cared for or they may have been abused or neglected in their first few years of life, and they require somewhat different nurturing to assure them that their new home is with their permanent (and new) family. Prospective parents must discuss these factors with social workers, psychologists, attorneys, pediatricians, or other professionals who can be sources of information helpful to their decision making (Kirby and Hardesty, 1998). Indeed, the concerns and complexities of contemporary adoption are such that a cover story in *U.S. News and World Report* in early 2001 was headlined "The Adoption Maze: More Couples Are Chasing Fewer Babies. The Experience Can Be Difficult, Dangerous, and Heartbreaking" (Clark and Shute, 2001).

> Adoption is at once a marvel of humanity and a social safety valve. It permits the infertile among us to share the deeply fulfilling, profoundly joyful experience of raising children. It offers a positive option for people who, for moral or economic or personal reasons, believe they can neither undergo an abortion nor parent a child. Most important, whatever it might accomplish for the adults in the picture, it provides a systematic opportunity for children to grow up in stable homes with loving parents. (Pertman, 2000, p. 8)

As true as this statement might be for people within the United States, it is probably an even more valid statement for biological parents in third world countries who feel unable to raise a child. For those who happily welcome the children into a family, and for the children involved, adoption truly is a marvel and a miracle.

The Biological Parents

Adoption policies change quickly on the international scene, sometimes quite unpredictably. In some countries, newborns are removed from their mothers without their consent and placed in orphanages for adoption for a substantial fee—a fee most often paid by Americans. In almost all countries, the prospective parents must meet several criteria or demands even before they are allowed to consider a specific child. That is in addition to conditions set by the Bureau of Citzenship and Immigration Services (BCIS) (to be discussed later in this chapter) and comparable services in other countries.

In the case of transracial or multicultural adoptions within this country, there are mixed reactions on the part of nonwhites about adoption of *their* children by whites (Schwartz, 2000). There is concern that the children will lose their African-American or Hispanic or Native American or Asian heritage, and that they will be lost to that community. To this end, there are laws encouraging adoption within the child's ethnic community of origin as well as on behalf of adoption rather than continued foster care. The Adoption and Safe Families Act of 1997, similar to its predecessor, the Multiethnic Placement Act of 1994 (amended in 1996), however, does not permit racial/ethnic differences to be considered in adoption.

Obviously, if a white parent adopts a biracial or other-ethnic child, the difference between parent and child will be readily apparent, and the parent will need to make appropriate explanations to the child early in the child's preelementary school years or when the child appears to become aware of the differences. It helps if the new family lives in a multicultural area where there may be enough of a mix of backgrounds that the child's difference from the adopting parents is not perceived as unusual (Babb and Laws, 1997). The difference is not as unique today in many communities as it might have been a generation ago, when there might have been no other nonwhite or multiethnic children in an elementary school except for the adoptee.

WHERE DO WE BEGIN?

Some people turn to the yellow pages of their local telephone directory and simply look up the numbers of adoption agencies or those listed as "facilitators." Others have friends or family members who know someone who might be able to help them find an adoptable child. Still others turn to the Internet with its thousands of Web sites dealing with adoption. Whichever route is taken, obviously the prospective parents need to verify credentials, know how the agency or individual negotiates the adoption between pregnant female and prospective parents, what legal requirements have to be met, and what costs are involved. They certainly must be aware that "buying" or "selling" a baby is illegal in every state, although payment of the mother's medical costs and of expenses related to the pregnancy is usually permitted.

According to the National Adoption Information Clearinghouse (2000), the costs of adoption can vary from virtually zero, in the case of some special needs adoptions via domestic public agencies, to

$25,000 to $30,000 in cases of independent adoption, whether domestic or international. These costs include agency fees for home study, attorney fees, advertising, birth-parent fees (usually restricted by state law), and additional fees to the State Department and possibly the government or an overseas agency in the case of foreign-country adoptions. Tax benefits and subsidies available to adopting parents may help offset some of these costs. In a nation where the Tenth Amendment protects states' rights, there is little national policy on adoption or the rights of adopted children, except those policies involving multicultural adoptions, as noted, or overseas adoptions, which are overseen by the Office of Children Issues of the U.S. Department of State. Hence, domestic adoption is subject to laws and practices that vary from state to state as well as within states.

As a cautionary example of why prospective parents need to know with whom they are dealing and under what regulations, one needs only to think of the twin newborns adopted—twice—with the "help" of an Internet facilitator who also knew which state has the least demanding residency requirements. Born in June 2000 to an interracial couple moving toward divorce, the twins were first placed with a couple in San Diego; a few months later, the facilitator re placed them with a British couple who were willing to pay her a higher fee. She then rushed the couple and the twins to Arkansas, which had a thirty-day residency requirement for surrendering parents as well as adoptive parents. Everyone lied about being a resident of the state, and the twins' adoption by the British couple was announced in December; they then rushed home to Wales. The San Diego couple sought to recover custody. By mid-January, the British government had intervened, removed the twins from their new home in Wales, and placed them in a foster home until their custody could be clarified. Their biological mother then said that she wanted them back; her soon-to-be-ex-husband, their father, said *he* wanted them; and the California couple still wanted them (though they subsequently withdrew their "claim"). Early in March 2001, the judge in Arkansas nullified the adoption because of all the perjury involved with regard to the residency requirement (Skoloff, 2001). The following month, the British courts ordered the twins' transfer back to the United States, to the custody of the court in St. Louis (Stange, 2001). At eight months of age, these little girls had been in at least four homes and under the care of probably a dozen people, and it appeared that no one was attending to the fact that, at this age, they were supposed to be developing trust in caretakers and building lasting attachment bonds with their "parents." Meanwhile, the adults involved, particularly the would-be parents, had the children they had quickly come to love ripped out of their lives, and their lives put in turmoil. This is not how anyone envisions adoption.

The lesson in this instance is to be extremely cautious in the choice of intermediary. A list of several legitimate agencies for domestic and international adoptions is included in the appendix to this book. It is also suggested that legal assistance be sought from a member of the American Academy of Adoption Attorneys, if only to be reasonably certain that the attorney is quite familiar with adoption laws and procedures here and abroad.

WHAT ARE OUR OPTIONS?

The traditional mode of adoption in the United States has been through a public social welfare agency, with the prospective parents undergoing intense inspection of every aspect of their lives as well as a home study, usually both before and after placement. The post-placement study meets state requirements regarding the care and welfare of the child in his or her new home. Biological parents do not have to experience such intrusions in their lives (Schwartz, 1996). A reviewer of Bernstein's *The Lost Children of Wilder* opened her review with a statement about *her* experience with New York's public adoption agencies. She was told that first she would have to serve as a foster parent, caring for "an abused or neglected child for 18 months" (Williams, 2001). From what she wrote, it would be *that* child she would be allowed to adopt if parental rights were terminated; if not, she would have to start a new cycle with a new foster child.

Independent adoption, often through a physician, an attorney, a clergyperson, or a private adoption agency, is an alternative to an agency's screening for acceptance as a prospective adoptive parent, although it is not legal in at least six states (National Adoption Information Clearinghouse, 2002). The availability of a "facilitator," who may or may not be a medical or legal professional, or of an advertisement by a pregnant woman seeking parents for her child-to-be, has increased in recent years, especially on the Internet, and great caution must be exercised in dealing with these unknown individuals. There may be some increased flexibility today even within agencies, certainly when it comes to removing children from prolonged foster care and finding them a permanent adoptive home, but the wait can still be long, the child found will more than likely *not* be a newborn—the first choice of most couples—and the ultimate choice may be between a special needs child and no child at all.

Special Needs Children

A special needs child is one who has been born with the effects of substance abuse or illness transmitted during the pregnancy, or who has genetic defects due to a problem gene or a mishap or neglect during pregnancy or at birth (see Chapter 5). The child may have a predicted short life span due to one of these problems (see Chapter 13), or have Down's syndrome, a sensory defect, or even a distorted or missing limb. In some cases, a child remained with the birth parent(s) after his or her arrival, but problems such as physical or emotional abuse may have occurred, with the result that the child was placed in foster care. This child may not become adoptable for a few years, by which time emotional and behavior problems may arise, making this child another with special needs. It is obviously of critical importance that the prospective adoptive parents be told everything that is known about the child's current and potential health or other problems (to the extent that they are known) and about the biological parents' medical histories, so that they are as aware as possible of the challenges they may have to meet in addition to those normally faced by parents (Kirby and Hardesty, 1998).

Older Children

Older children, possibly even in their early or middle school years, are yet another group seeking permanent homes. These may be domestic or international adoptions, and they pose a different set of challenges than infants. Developing trust in new parents after several years of being moved from one home to another, or after having been in an orphanage with multiple changing caretakers, is often difficult for an eight- or nine-year-old. These children may be behind in learning skills because of neglect or lack of opportunity, so that this becomes a problem for prospective parents as well as a source of teasing by peers in the new community. Extensive screening to determine the nature of any problems they may have is also recommended (Kirby and Hardesty, 1998). Prospective parents should also ask whether there are any siblings who may have been raised elsewhere, and whether it is feasible and/or desirable to adopt the sibling(s) as well (see Chapter 11).

Transcultural Adoption

Children with a multiracial background may or may not be welcomed in their biological families and communities. If they are part Native American, there may be intensive efforts to keep them within the tribe because of the dual concern that the children will lose their ethnic identity and the tribe will lose the renewal and strength that the younger generation brings. This concern resulted in passage of the Indian Child Welfare Act of 1978, which gave first preference to adoption of such children by Native Americans (Howard, 1984; Schwartz, 1996). The National Association of Black Social Workers (NABSW) has long sought similar preferential treatment, alleging that the adoption of black children by white parents is injurious to the children's development, although there is only mixed support for that view in studies of such children postadoption (Schwartz, 1996). In many cases, for example, black children were in the care of white foster parents but then could not be adopted by them because of pressures for placement with black parents (see Chapter 13). However, as noted earlier, to prevent the use of race as the sole criterion in arranging adoptive (or even foster care) placements, the Multiethnic Placement Act of 1994 was passed, prohibiting agencies that receive federal funds from such a practice (Schwartz, 2000), with the law's provisions clarified and strengthened by the Interethnic Adoption Provisions of the Small Business Job Protection Act of 1996 (National Adoption Information Clearinghouse, 2000). The Adoption and Safe Families Act of 1997 has the same provision.

If not adopted in their own community, these children may then become eligible for adoption by people of other backgrounds—more often by middle- or upper-class whites than by any other group (Pertman, 2000). Depending on the nature of the community to which they then move, they may or may not find acceptance by their peers and the surrounding adults. They have only to look in the mirror to know that they do not resemble their parents, which may or may not distress them. (If you think that there are too many "or"s included here, be advised that flat generalities cannot be made regarding outcomes because of the number of variables that contribute to them.)

The final option is to seek a child overseas.

International Adoption

Pearl Buck, a well-known twentieth-century author and winner of the Nobel Prize for Literature in 1938, was a leader in promoting adoption of children from other countries—from China initially, in her case. An adoptive mother herself, she founded Welcome House in 1949 in response to the unwillingness of American adoption agencies to place Asian and multiracial children. She also established a foundation to support Asian-American children who were not eligible for adoption (Conn, 1996). A pioneering program, Welcome House is still an active agency for international adoptions and has expanded its activities to several other Asian countries as well as Romania and Russia. Other agencies also arrange adoptions in Asia today, as well as in countries of the former Soviet bloc and in Latin America. The number of orphan children granted immigrant visas to the United States so that they could be adopted here went from 8,481 in 1991 to 19,237 in 2001, with the majority of children being female and age four years or younger (National Adoption Information Clearinghouse, 2002). In 2002, the number of immigrant visas issued to orphans coming to the United States exceeded 20,000 (U.S. Department of State, 2003).

In all of these countries, from Peru to Guatemala to Romania to China, Cambodia, and Vietnam, the rules relevant to adoption can change almost without notice to anyone, especially the prospective adoptive parents who may have traveled thousands of miles and spent tens of thousands of dollars for the opportunity to adopt a child. Elizabeth Bartholet (1993), a Harvard lawyer, has described some of the bureaucratic snarls with which she was confronted in Peru. Others have written of the malnutrition and poor care that children may have received in their home country (Verhulst, Althaus, and Versluis-Den Bieman, 1990; Wardle, 1990). A colleague who had been in Romania in February 2001 told of seeing young children living in sewers there. Indeed, they were shown in the sewers as well as begging on the streets on *20/20* in June of that year (Walters, 2001). Adoptive parents too often have not been given full information about resulting problems, both medical and psychological. Conditions in orphanages are often deplorable and certainly not conducive to what Americans consider normal child development.

On the part of the adoptees, children approaching school age or older have to try to put their earlier experiences aside, learn a new language, bond with new adults and possibly siblings, and adjust to a totally strange environment (Schwartz, 2000) (see Chapter 11). This is a daunting challenge for them and for those who adopt them. In addition, many are puzzled by their biological parents' apparent lack of interest in them.

Special needs are a concern with international as well as domestic adoptions, for many of the children in orphanages in third world countries, or even those being adopted directly from their biological parents, similarly have a variety of special needs about which the adopting parents need to be informed (Quarles and Brodie, 1998). Indeed, Jeffreys (1996/1997) has urged that medical screening of international adoptees be made mandatory because of the prevalence of lead poisoning, HIV, hepatitis, intestinal diseases, tuberculosis, and other conditions of which, at minimum, the prospective parents should be aware (see Chapter 9). Unfortunately, some of the overseas sources have not been as forthcoming with accurate and honest information about the children as they should be. Prospective parents, anxious as they may be to adopt a child, really need to be sure that their intermediary, whether an agency or an individual, obtains all pertinent information about the child so that there are as few negative surprises as possible to threaten the development of family bonds.

Although there can be many difficulties to surmount in international adoptions, the arguments for taking this route include the relative lack of risk of a birth mother changing her mind, seeking to reclaim the child, or reappearing in the child's life. This feature alone makes this type of adoption more attractive to many couples (Salzer, 1999). That is not to say that the birth mother may not change her mind *before* the adoptive parents receive permission to take the child to the United States, but it is rare afterward. For some would-be parents, there is also a strong feeling of doing a good deed (i.e., literally saving a child from a terrible fate) that enhances the adoption experience (see Chapters 4, 6, and 13).

One barrier that *has* been reduced for children being adopted from other countries is the current more rapid acquisition of American citizenship, thanks to the Child Citizenship Act of 2000 (U.S. Department of State, 2001). Foreign-born children under age eighteen residing with their adoptive parent(s) in the United States now automatically become U.S. citizens as soon as the adoption decree is final. In addition, the State Department circulates information regarding practices in the source nations overseas, with warnings of a variety of potential difficulties, as appropriate. As of early June 2002, for example, the State Department was warning U.S. citizens that they should not pursue adoptions in Cambodia or Mongolia until further notice because of problems affecting adoption *within* those countries, and that Laos was not permitting external adoptions. Legal requirements that have to be met both here and abroad are also clearly stated, either in print or on the State Department's Web site (www.travel.state.gov/int'ladoption. html).

Other difficulties regarding overseas adoptions may be reduced once the United States has in place the means to implement provisions of the 1993 Hague Convention on Intercountry Adoption, probably by 2004. Although the United States was one of the countries participating in the negotiations that resulted in the convention, Congress did not agree to sign it until September 2000, a decision approved by President Clinton the following month (Office of Children's Issues, 2000).

OTHER CONSIDERATIONS IN CREATING A FAMILY

Clearly, anyone seeking to adopt one or more children has to be prepared for a number of unanticipated events in the development of a family relationship. Frankly, with respect to the child's personality and development, much depends on the age of the child being adopted and the child's prenatal and early childhood experiences. Help can be obtained from a variety of professionals and agencies as needed, both before and after the adoption. Some of the potential difficulties with which the new family may need assistance have already been discussed.

There are also ways in which the background of multiracial/multicultural and international adoptees can be used to enrich the family.

Introduction of elements of the child's background, through photographs of the child's home country or even the biological family if available, rituals incorporating the child's native culture, or interaction with others sharing the child's background can become an integral part of the family's life together (Lieberman and Bufferd, 1999). This is amply illustrated in many chapters in this book. Parents who have adopted children from the same geographical area may meet on a regular or irregular basis, in effect becoming a mutual support group as well as a group in which the children can interact with others who have a similar background. It may be that, as the child becomes old enough to understand the experience, the family can travel to Guatemala or Russia or Korea to become acquainted with the land and people of the child's origins. Many families have done this (see, particularly, Chapter 8).

Most important, perhaps, is that the adopting parents make it very clear they have a full mental and emotional commitment to the child, no matter where the child's roots may have been. This is true in all adoptions, not just multicultural and international ones.

INTRODUCING PERSONAL STORIES

Ongoing research with adoptive families described in Chapter 2 provides a broad-based and long-term context for the individual stories that follow, wherein adoptive parents discuss the pleasures and pains they have experienced in adopting children of a background different from their own. These author-parents, some of whom have chosen to write under pseudonyms, have had a wide variety of experiences. In one chapter, the adopted daughter has added her thoughts; in another, the biological children and maternal grandmother have contributed other perspectives. Hopefully, readers who are contemplating international or nontraditional adoption, as well as professionals working with members of such special adoptive families, will become better informed about the cautions and benefits of these less than traditional adoptions by reading and thinking about these narratives. Every family, biological or adoptive in origin, has its stories; these are unusually rich.

REFERENCES

Babb, L. A. and Laws, R. (1997). *Adoption and advocating for the special needs child.* Westport, CT: Greenwood Publishing.

Bartholet, E. (1993). *Family bonds: Adoption and the politics of parenting.* New York: Houghton Mifflin.

Broyde, M. (1998). Cloning people: A Jewish law analysis of the issues. *Connecticut Law Review, 30,* 503.

Clark, K. and Shute, N. (2001). The adoption maze. *U.S. News & World Report,* March 12, pp. 60-69.

Conn, P. (1996). Pearl Sydenstricker Buck, 1892-1973. Accessed online: <www.pearlbuck.org/psbi/PearlSBuck/about.asp>.

Diamond, R., Kezur, D., Meyers, M., Scharf, C. N., and Weinshel, M. (1999). *Couple therapy for infertility.* New York: Guilford Press.

Howard, M. (1984). Transracial adoption: Analysis of the best interests standard. *Notre Dame Law Review, 59,* 503-555.

Jeffreys, D. P. (1996/1997). Intercountry adoption: A need for mandatory medical screening. *Journal of Law and Health, 11,* 243.

Kirby, K. M. and Hardesty, P. H. (1998). Evaluating older pre-adoptive foster children. *Professional Psychology, 19,* 428-436.

Lieberman, C. A. and Bufferd, R. K. (1999). *Creating ceremonies: Innovative ways to meet adoption challenges.* Phoenix, AZ: Zeig, Tucker, and Theisen, Inc.

Molock, S. D. (1999). Racial, cultural, and religious issues in infertility counseling. In L. H. Burns and S. N. Covington (Eds.), *Infertility counseling: A comprehensive handbook for clinicians* (pp. 249-265). New York: Parthenon Publishing.

National Adoption Information Clearinghouse (2000). Accessed online: <www.calib.com/naic/pubs>.

National Adoption Information Clearinghouse (2002). Accessed online: <www.calib.com/naic/pubs>.

Office of Children's Issues, U.S. Department of State (2000). The 1993 Hague Intercountry Adoption Convention: Status of and concepts underlying U.S. federal implementing legislation. Accessed online: <travel.state.gov/status_concepts.html>.

Oz, S. J. (1995). Genetic mother vs. surrogate mother: Which mother does the law recognize? A comparison of Jewish law, American law, and England's law. *Touro International Law Review, 6,* 438.

Pertman, A. (2000). *Adoption nation: How the adoption revolution is transforming America.* New York: Basic Books.

Povarsky, C. (1998). Regulating advanced reproductive technologies: A comparative analysis of Jewish and American law. *University of Toledo Law Review, 29,* 409.

Quarles, C. S. and Brodie, J. H. (1998). Primary care of international adoptees. *American Family Physician, 58* (December), 2025-2032, 2039-2040.

Salzer, L. P. (1999). Adoption after infertility. In L. H. Burns and S. N. Covington (Eds.), *Infertility counseling: A comprehensive handbook for clinicians* (pp. 391-409). New York: Parthenon Publishing.

Schwartz, L. L. (1987). Surrogate motherhood I: Responses to infertility. *American Journal of Family Therapy, 15,* 158-162.

Schwartz, L. L. (1991). *Alternatives to infertility: Is surrogacy the answer?* New York: Brunner/Mazel.

Schwartz, L. L. (1996). Adoptive families: Are they nonnormative? In M. Harway (Ed.), *Treating the changing family: Handling normative and unusual events* (pp. 97-114). New York: John Wiley.

Schwartz, L. L. (2000). Adoption: Parents who choose their children and their options. In F. W. Kaslow (Ed.), *Handbook of Couples and Family Forensics* (pp. 23-42). New York: John Wiley.

Skoloff, B. (2001). British pair's adoption of U.S. twins nullified. *The Philadelphia Inquirer,* March 7, p. A2.

Stange, J. (2001). Twins in custody case back in U.S. *The Philadelphia Inquirer,* April 20, p. A10.

U.S. Department of State (2001). Child Citizenship Act of 2000. Accessed online: <travel.state.gov/childcit.html>, February 26.

U.S. Department of State (2003). Immigrant visas issued to orphans coming to the U.S. Accessed online: <http://travel.state.gov/orphan_numbers.html>.

Verhulst, F. C., Althaus, M., and Versluis-Den Bieman, H. J. M. (1990). Problem behavior in international adoptees: II. Age at placement. *Journal of the American Academy of Child and Adolescent Psychiatry, 29,* 2104-2111.

Walters, B. (2001). Children for sale. *20/20,* ABC-TV Network, June 8.

Wardle, F. (1990). Endorsing children's differences: Meeting the needs of minority children. *Young Children, 45*(5), 44-46.

Williams, P. J. (2001). A sad cycle of bounces in foster care. *The New York Times,* March 29, p. E-7.

Chapter 2

Welcome Home: From the Perspective of Research on International Adoption

Paul A. Lipton
Sanno Zack
Stephen A. Petrill
Jeffery Flanagan
Kirby Deater-Deckard

What is a family? How are cultural traditions passed down through the generations? How do parents raise their children to develop a healthy sense of self and identity? These questions, although meaningful in all families, are thrust to the forefront in adoptive families, especially when children come from a different cultural and/or ethnic background than their adoptive parents.

The popular and psychological literature is filled with reports examining how well internationally or transethnically adopted children "do" after adoption—examining such outcomes as psychological adjustment, attachment to parents, and academic success. Surprisingly, very little attention has been paid to the perspective of adoptive parents. How do adoptive parents feel about raising a biologically unrelated child, and what particular issues do they think about? In turn, how do these feelings and attitudes affect the child? How do the children affect the parents?

Our goal in this chapter is to describe the experiences of international and transethnic adoptive families who participated in our research study. These reports are meant to highlight some of the important issues that parents have expressed to us concerning the process of

This project was supported by a grant from the Society for the Psychological Study of Social Issues and a National Science Foundation Collaborative Research Award to Stephen A. Petrill (BCS-9907811) and Kirby Deater-Deckard (BCS-9907860).

preparing for and raising a child of another ethnicity. This chapter is organized into three main sections. The first section describes our interests as researchers studying transethnic adoption and provides a description of the adoptive families with whom we have been working. The second section describes the methods we used in our study. The third section presents selected responses from these families, detailing the various aspects of their adoption experience. It is our hope that this information from the adoptive parents' experience will be useful to prospective parents interested in transethnic adoption as well as those families who have already come together through adoption.

THE NORTHEAST-NORTHWEST COLLABORATIVE ADOPTION PROJECTS (N²CAP)

For the past three years, we have been conducting the Northeast-Northwest Collaborative Adoption Project (N²CAP), which at present includes 1,489 adopted children and their families. Our interest as researchers was to establish a large sample of adoptive families so that we might identify environmental influences associated with cognitive ability, academic achievement, emotional development, and behavioral development. The adoptive family, because the parents and children are genetically unrelated, provides a unique opportunity to directly assess aspects of the family environment that contribute to similarities among family members. As part of this larger project, we also asked parents numerous questions about why they chose to adopt as well as their attitudes toward international adoption. Thus, while the parents in our study have taught us a great deal about international adoption, this component of our study is part of a larger, more general, research effort. In addition, our interaction with such a large number of families who have experienced the adoption process affords us a unique perspective on the subject of international adoption, albeit not the result of firsthand personal experience. Finally, although our sample is large, it is also self-selected. Thus, we cannot know if the responses in our study are generalizable to all adoptive parents or are representative of a subset of adoptive parents. What we, therefore, report here is a reflection of the experiences described to us by the parents who have had personal experience adopting children from outside of the United States.

Demographics of the Sample

The N^{2}CAP is a continuing project and data are still being collected. The information that follows is, therefore, from our latest analysis. The project is based at the Pennsylvania State University (northeast site) and the University of Oregon (northwest site). Of the parents in this sample of families, 95 percent identified themselves as white. In contrast, 66 percent of the children were reportedly from nonwhite ethnic backgrounds, including Asian, African American, Latino, and other ethnicities. On average, the children in this sample began living with their adoptive families at the age of one year.

The parents in this sample are highly educated. More than 80 percent of the parents graduated with at least a four-year college degree, whereas in the general population that number is lower, at about 50 percent. In addition, approximately 40 percent of the parents completed some type of graduate or professional school, whereas in the general population the number is closer to 25 percent (U.S. Department Education, NCES, 2001).

A significant percentage of the mothers and fathers within the current N^{2}CAP sample are from dual-earner families; 96 percent of the fathers work outside the home, and nearly 70 percent of the mothers reported working at a job outside the home. It is possible that with a large number of single parents this number would be artificially inflated. This, however, is not the case in this sample, given that 85 percent of mothers reported being married or cohabitating, and 98 percent reported that they live with either their spouse or partner. Parental occupations span the spectrum, including many physicians, engineers, consultants, nurses, architects, managers, midlevel employees, teachers, social workers, dance instructors, and editors. In addition, a significant number of mothers did report that they stay at home to care for their children.

Measures

Structure

Information was collected from the families in the N^{2}CAP in two stages. The demographic information previously reported was collected as part of the first stage of the N^{2}CAP. In the second stage, parents filled out three separate questionnaires. The first one, titled "Family Questionnaire," asked parents to report their reasons for adopting and their feelings about child rearing and general educational issues (Rescorla et al., 1990; Schaefer and Edgerton, 1985). The second questionnaire, titled "Individual Questionnaire," was devoted to measuring the emotional, social, cognitive, and behavioral adjustment of each child (Child Behavior Checklist [CBCL]: Achenbach, 1991; Strengths and Difficulties Questionnaire [SDQ]: Goodman, 1997), in addition to the parents' feelings toward each child (Parent Feelings Questionnaire [PFQ]: Deater-Deckard, 1996). No interviews were conducted with these children, though interactions between the child and one of the adoptive parents were observed. The third questionnaire, titled "International Adoption Questionnaire" (Tessler, Gamache, and Liu, 1996), was designed for parents who had adopted a child born in another country. This questionnaire was used to assess how the parents prepared for the process of transethnic adoption, their attitudes toward the birth culture of their adopted child, and their attitudes about American culture. At the time these questionnaires were administered, the average age of the children was approximately six years old. The range of ages was considerable given that many of the families had completed the adoption proceedings several years prior to participation in the project. These children averaged one year old at the time they were adopted.

Categorization

Each completed Family and International Adoption Questionnaire holds responses to nearly 150 questions. Each question asks about a very specific feeling, desire, attitude, or belief within one of several general areas related to the adoption experience. For example, in one instance, the parents were asked to rate the level of importance of having their child learn about American values and traditions, whereas in another they were asked about their feelings toward a child's obedience to authority. Each of these questions provides a certain amount of information in its own right. Yet analyzing the impact of each individual question and devising a theoretical framework complete with interpretations based on the individual responses is unreasonable. Many of the individual questions, in fact, overlap in subject area. For example, several questions from the International Adoption Questionnaire address the issue of the language of the child's birth country. It is certainly interesting to know how a parent feels about his or her child being able to write his or her own name in his or her birth language. However, it is arguably more valuable to get a sense of the broader picture, that is, how the parents feel about their child acquiring the ability to communicate in his or her birth language. With this in mind, sets of questions were initially grouped together based on the parents' responses. These groupings were then validated using theoretical and statistical methods. The result of this procedure was that thirty-three categories emerged covering the different aspects of the adoption process. The following section outlines the different questions that were asked and the resulting categories into which those individual questions were collapsed.

THE QUESTIONS: THE FAMILY QUESTIONNAIRE

Reasons, Education, and Child Rearing

The Family Questionnaire addressed two issues. The first consideration was the reason people adopt. A popular conception of why individuals decide to adopt is that the prospective parents are infertile. Is this generally the case, or do other factors influence their decision? To answer this and other questions, we asked all of the parents within the N^2CAP sample a series of questions addressing their motivation for adoption:

> Did the parents feel pressure from their families or friends to have a child?
> Were they ensuring an emotional or financial support system for when they got older?
> Did the infertility factor enter into their decision to adopt?

The second broad consideration in the Family Questionnaire involved parenting, child rearing, and thoughts about education. The parents were asked to rate the level of importance of the following representative statements:

Children should always obey their parents.

Teachers should discipline children all the same.

Children have a right to their own point of view, and to expressing it.

Preparation for the future is more important for children than enjoying the present.

The major goal of education is to put basic information into the minds of children.

Responses to these statements were combined and resulted in the following general categories: authority and obedience, fair treatment, children unruly, right to opinions, pressure, teacher and home environment, and child education.

International Adoption

As was mentioned earlier in this chapter, adopting and raising a child from a different cultural and ethnic background is a multifaceted process. The adopted child, as he or she becomes more aware of his or her environment, realizes the difference between himself or herself and friends and parents. The child might start to ask questions about his or her birth country and sometimes show an interest in a further exploration of this original world (i.e., the birth culture). How the adoptive parents deal with this interest, prepare for these questions, and express their own views may have a considerable impact on the manner in which the child incorporates these new details and identifies with either the adopted or birth culture. For example, one research group has reported that the way parents describe the racial characteristics of their child directly relates to the child's view of his or her race (McRoy et al., 1982). It is understandable that this consideration is often overlooked by parents given that biological families generally are not faced with the subject of which cultural values to present or how to present them to their children. Biological family members often look similar to one another and share many aspects of their personalities and character traits by virtue of their shared genetic and socialization histories. This may not be the case for some families who have adopted internationally; certainly, the child is unrelated genetically, and he or she may look different from the adoptive parents. The International Adoption Questionnaire, therefore, attempts to address this by asking about specific attitudes and feelings regarding multicultural diversity.

Preparation

First the parents were asked how they prepared for the adoption. Parents were asked to indicate whether they attended parent support or counseling groups, talked with friends and family, visited their child's birth country, or obtained materials from the adoption agency about their child's birth culture. Second, they were asked about their experience of the adoption process. A sample of statements follows:

> I was prepared mentally for raising a child of another ethnicity.
> I feel it is most important to develop my transethnic adoptee's sense of ethnic identity.
> I often seek advice from an individual or organization from the same ethnic group as my child.

Third, their attitudes regarding ethnically diverse relationships were assessed by asking about child participation in groups or organizations with other members of the child's birth culture and by asking parents to indicate how important it is that the child be enrolled in a racially integrated school. In more general terms, we tried to assess the scope and to identify the specific methods of the parents' mental and experiential preparation for their transethnic adoption experience.

Attitudes Toward Birth Culture

Next the parents were asked to report their attitudes about multicultural diversity within the home. On the one hand, these questions allowed us to gauge the parents' level of interest in providing multicultural opportunities for their children. On the other hand, they revealed the potential conflict between the parents' desire for their children to incorporate their adopted culture and their desire not to abandon their birth culture. This raises what may be one of the most significant issues faced by parents of adopted children: How do I foster a sense of my family's cultural identity while valuing my child's cultural and ethnic heritage? Thus, to characterize more specifically how the parents felt about their adopted child's relation to his or her birth culture, we sought responses to the following representative statements:

> Child learns about values and traditions of birth country.
> Child becomes bilingual with native language.
> Child visits birth country as a teenager.
> Child learns to love his/her birth country.

Responses were reduced to the following subcategories: exposure, communication, travel to the adopted child's birth country, and ethnic pride.

Attitudes Toward American Culture

Regarding the extent to which the parents wanted their children to experience, or incorporate, aspects of American culture, the following statements were presented:

> Child dresses like other American children.
> Child is proud of his or her American heritage.
> Child goes to "sleepovers" at a friend's house.
> Child learns the American attitude of valuing self-esteem.
> Child visits Statue of Liberty.
> Child learns Mother Goose nursery rhymes.

These were the resulting subcategories: American commercial culture, civic pride, extrafamilial relations, parents' and American values, exposure to national treasures, American stories.

SURVEY FINDINGS

It is worth noting that while we examined overall trends in these surveys, the resulting interpretations are based on statistical averages. The experiences of individual parents could and do vary, sometimes considerably.

Reasons for Adopting

As mentioned earlier, there are several possible motivations for deciding to adopt a child. As expected, infertility is an important motivation for adoption. However, approximately one-third of all respondents reported that fertility was not an issue. Approximately one-third of the parents felt it was important to pass on their values to another generation. Of parents, 23 percent reported that they wanted to give their child another sibling, whereas 28 percent reported a desire to provide opportunities that they themselves never had. Also, a majority (68 percent) simply wished to have the parenting experience. As one family reported, "Once we realized being *parents* was important to us, not necessarily the birth process, it was easier to make the leap." Finally, the vast majority did not report any significant pressure from family or friends. Thus, individuals interested in adoption considered a variety of issues prior to making their decision.

Rearing and Education

The issue of child rearing and education was addressed so that we could generate a broad understanding of the parents and their general attitudes. The responses of this particular group of parents reflected a less-than-enthusiastic embrace of authority. Though their general feelings toward obedience reflected a mild agreement that children should obey parents and teachers, their responses tended toward ambivalence when faced with words such as "loyalty," "always," and "absolute." In the case of dealing with children both at home and in school, the parents generally preferred to have their sibling children treated differently from one another, i.e., as the individuals they are. Many parents with more than one child emphasized their children's differences in a free-response section, detailing each child's "unique character" and adding statements such as "Our children are as different as night and day."

When it comes to behavior, this group of parents felt that children are generally well behaved and do not require constant supervision or careful treatment. They did not feel it was important that their children always be busy with schoolwork or engaged in some productive extracurricular enterprise. They felt it was perfectly reasonable behavior for their children to disagree with them or with other adults. In fact, the parents felt strongly about their children having their own points of view and feeling comfortable expressing them.

When asked the open-ended question "What kind of job would you like your child to have?", the vast majority of parents reported, "Any job that makes my child happy." Nevertheless, this group of parents held high educational expectations for their children, with many parents indicating that their children would eventually attend college or pursue a graduate or professional degree.

These parents felt that education does not and should not take place only in the school. They expressed the sentiment that what their children learn at home has a considerable impact on their performance at school. In addition, they reported that it is reasonable for teachers to be concerned with, and inquire about, what goes on at home. As far as the methods by which a child learns best, for example, rote memorization or hands-on experience, and the kinds of basic information children are supposed to learn in school, no "typical" pattern emerged; the parents differed in their responses. One parent expressed this about her son:

> He is a self-driven individual with wonderful focus—a clinical mind—which analyzes things with great focus/concentration. He is his own wonderful *self*-instructor! He chooses to be alone, is not excluded as a loner.

Another parent described the following nightly ritual about her son:

> He is an excellent reader. After we read to him in the evening, he often takes a book to bed. He is very interested in foreign languages. We've taught him a little Spanish and French. He's always asking for more. Wish I had more time and knowledge.

The viewpoints of this particular group of parents suggested that their methods of child rearing did not include strict adherence to authority within the school and at home. In the context of our research interests with the N^{2}CAP, these child-rearing attitudes may ultimately prove informative as we try to understand how the child's experience of identity development relates to his or her parents' feelings about that process.

Preparation

The two most common means of preparation for the adoption experience were to gather information about the child's birth culture from the adoption agency and to discuss this issue with family and friends. About 58 percent of the parents also attended parent support sessions and counseling groups. A small number (about one-quarter) reported that they had visited the adoptee's birth country as a means to prepare for the adoption. One mother shared, "I enjoyed traveling to our daughter's birth country and feel it is important for parents to go to their child's birth country. It broadened my cultural perspective." Overall it appears that the parents in this group made attempts to learn about and understand the impact of raising a child born outside of the United States. In fact, a couple of parents raised the issue that our questions regarding ethnicity, heritage, and culture forced a false dichotomy. Their child, they said, is "genetically" one thing, culturally another. The father said the child was adopted at four months of age, and so "he is an American of Korean and European descent. Many of your questions assume some sort of dissociation between him and his ethnicity and him and his parents (us)." Other families felt comfortable identifying all family members as "Asian American," "African American," or "Hispanic American."

One might gather from their attempts to familiarize themselves with the adoption process that the parents would report a generally positive experience. Indeed, their reports supported this assumption, with nearly 65 percent very satisfied. Of the parents, 90 percent thought that they were generally prepared mentally to raise a child of another ethnicity. As many as 80 percent reported that the process had been easier than expected. For some, however, the technical and financial aspects of the adoption process sometimes proved very difficult and included problems with adoption agencies, long waiting periods, and time-consuming paperwork. Wait time from initiation to bringing the child home ranged considerably, with some families receiving their child within five or six months and others waiting as long as four or five years. One father described the frustration of the waiting process: "The hardest part was the wait after all our paperwork was sent. I kept thinking of [our daughter] sitting in the orphanage while our dossier took seven months to go through the courts." In general, parents in this sample seemed to have a clear sense of the importance of a good fit between family and agency. One mother explained, "Due to my adoption agency, my adoption was not difficult. Communication between agency and client is very important [as is] accessibility of agency and client—this is rare, though."

Two questions in the questionnaires asked the parents how they felt about developing or emphasizing their adopted child's sense of transethnic or American identity. There was general agreement on the importance of developing the adopted child's sense of his or her original ethnic identity, with nearly 80 percent expressing this sentiment. The same number of parents reported that it was also important to develop their child's sense of American identity. Finally, a similar percentage believed that it was important to emphasize both aspects of identity equally.

Decisions regarding how and when to discuss issues of identity with transethnic adopted children may appear complex. One mother explained:

> I often wonder if and when and how I should explain the adoption process to my children who are two and four. They both know they are from China. I worry sometimes if they will ever experience discrimination in this country. I never want them to be hurt. So far we have not had that experience, although we get many questions about where they are from.

One way to envision developing or emphasizing a child's sense of ethnic identity might be to help the child foster relationships with other individuals of the same ethnicity. A second approach would be to enroll the child in a racially integrated school or to live in a racially integrated community. Many of the parents expressed an interest in these alternatives, thus favoring an opportunity for the child to experience, firsthand, life in a community that included certain aspects of his or her own birth culture.

Cultural Attitudes

If parents adopt a child born in another country, often they find themselves confronted with a language barrier. Since the vast majority of children adopted in N²CAP were infants, most parents did not encounter the problem of speaking a different language than their child. However, as the child gets older, he or she may develop an interest in learning the language of his or her birth culture. The parents in our study responded with varying degrees of interest in either this idea or the prospect of being able to communicate with their child in that language. A further exploration of this topic may provide a better appreciation for these diverse attitudes and whether they reflect a desire not to pressure the child into learning a particular language, or whether the parents think that learning the language is not going to be a valuable experience. One of our questions did, however, ask parents how they felt about their adopted child learning a foreign language other than that of his or her birth country. Interestingly, this option was viewed as more important than being bilingual or able to write or learn words and phrases in the language of the child's birth country.

Another method of exposing the child to his or her birth culture is to have an in-home child care provider of the same ethnicity as the child. Few parents in this study were interested in this alternative. Other methods might include making foods, playing music, and reading stories from the child's birth country, as well as learning about the history and traditions of the child's birth culture. Again, no clear consensus emerged regarding how the parents intended to introduce their adopted child to his or her birth culture. On average, parents were moderately interested in exposing their adopted child to these basic aspects of the child's birth culture. Possibly the parents in this study have approached the question of how to engender a sense of ethnic identity in their adopted child in ways that differ from one family to another. Though many parents expressed a desire to foster their adopted child's sense of ethnic identity, the scope and specificity of our questions may not have provided the parents with the means to elaborate clearly their intentions. As a result, we are not able to characterize a common or typical approach toward fostering a sense of ethnic pride within these transethnic adoptive families.

We also examined parents' attitudes toward American culture. Exposure to American commercial culture, such as visiting Disneyland, having dolls or action figures, and seeing Disney movies, did not rate high on the parents' list of important values. The parents were generally noncommittal as far as having their adopted child learn American children's stories and visit American monuments. The parents were, however, fairly keen on their adopted child forming relationships outside the family with friends at school and friends from diverse ethnicities. In addition, the parents thought it was quite important that their adopted child develop a sense of civic pride, for example, learning the Pledge of Allegiance, being proud of his or her American heritage, and celebrating holidays such as the Fourth of July. These responses were consistent with the parents' attitudes about developing their adopted child's sense of American identity.

The Children

As mentioned earlier, one of our goals at the start of the N²CAP was to understand the transmission of cultural traditions and the interactions through which parents foster a healthy sense of self and identity in their adopted children. The age at which most of the children in this study were adopted precludes an analysis of the children's perceptions of their immediate environment with respect to their parents' attitudes and parenting practices. Therefore, through a set of additional questionnaires we asked the parents about their perceptions of their children's behavior and development.

A preliminary analysis of this information yielded the following observations. On the whole, the children in the N²CAP appeared fairly well adjusted behaviorally and emotionally. The most significant determinant of problem behaviors appears to stem from the age at which the children were placed into their adoptive homes. As the child's age of placement increases, he or she is more likely to demonstrate hyperactive behavior and other adjustment problems. The earlier a child is placed into his or her adoptive home, the better the chance that he or she will score higher on tests measuring IQ. Finally, mothers of children placed at younger ages demonstrated a more positive affect toward their adopted children.

Since we have not yet had the opportunity to explore the issue of identity development in this sample of transethnic adoptive families, we plan to continue the study to evaluate over time the role of parents and the children themselves in the children's development. Finally, another question we are interested in exploring is whether the attitudes of the parents vary according to the developmental stage of their adopted child. It is conceivable that some parents may become more interested in diverse cultures as they experience their child's exploration of his or her birth culture.

SUMMARY AND CONCLUDING REMARKS

In many respects, families participating in the N²CAP study represent a range of diverse experiences with adoption. It is still possible, however, that our survey results may not be representative of all adoptive families. Since participation was voluntary, it is possible that only families who enjoyed the experience responded.

Our sample included single mothers, homosexual and heterosexual partners, couples who adopted multiple children, and those who adopted a single child, as well as families with both biological and adopted children. Some families adopted internationally and others adopted domestically. Some families adopted children with special needs. Yet despite these differences, a number of common themes emerged. Parents were offered space on the questionnaires to report "anything else you would like to tell us." Many families chose to do so, and comments ranged from descriptions of the adoption process to details of the adopted child's personality. Although transethnic adoption can certainly present challenges, when given the opportunity parents focused on joys and trials that are common for all parents.

The most striking aspect of these responses was the overwhelmingly positive view that parents took of their adoption experience. "Becoming a parent has been the best experience of my life," wrote more than one mother or father. Children were described over and over as "the joy of our lives" and "precious gifts." Parents poured out pages of detail describing their children's warmth, intelligence, artistic ability, energy, passion, humor, charm, beauty, compassion, and a host of other strengths. Many families also reported that the addition of the child caused a deepening and strengthening of the adopting couple's relationship and helped each parent grow as an individual:

> I also feel that I am a better person because of my parenting role and experience. There is no question that the most important job/role in life is to be a parent, and that is also the most challenging and demanding (and the one you get the least training and preparation for!).

Not everything was easy, but parents in this study seemed to find more to celebrate than to complain about. Summed up one father, "Our lives have certainly changed since we adopted two children in a fourteen-month span! I don't think life has ever been so stressful for me, yet at the same time my life has never been so rich."

A number of families remarked on the challenges of the adoption process itself, yet many of these same families also commented on the benefits of participating in such a procedure:

> The adoption process was long and arduous, yet it really made [us] do some soul-searching as to why we want children and how we will raise our children. I have always thought that all families would be better off if they had to go through the process before having children.

A few families told stories of greater challenges, including coping with their child's disability or health problems, juggling working and parenting, or grappling with the financial challenges of being a single parent. One family who undertook a domestic adoption reported the following harrowing story:

> The adoption process put us through every test possible. Starting with having a little boy first. And the birth mother changing her mind. Thought we would never make it through that. Five weeks later [our daughter] came to live with us. When picking up [our daughter], the state lost the paperwork and [we] had to wait five weeks to leave the state. Living out of motels with a newborn child until the money ran out.

Yet even this family reported that the experience "turned out great in the end" and at the time of completing their questionnaires they were in the process of internationally adopting a second child. More than a few parents commented that their positive experience with their first adoption had prompted them to initiate a second. Wrote one mother, "I love being my children's mother as much as and more than I knew I would. I only wish time and circumstances made it practical for me to adopt three more!"

We think most parents would agree that adopting a child is a unique experience and one that rarely, if ever, leaves a family unchanged. The experience of transethnic adoption brings to families a full gamut of emotions. "Our adoption was fantastic, scary, exhilarating, and nerve-wracking from beginning to end," shared one mother.

Above all else, however, families in this study reported that the adoption experience had been a strongly positive one:

> Having a child is an important way of re-remembering what is really important in this life. It added much more to my life experience than I ever imagined possible. . . . Our children are the best things that have come into our lives. We are a complete family now.

REFERENCES

Achenbach, T. M. (1991). *Integrative guide for the 1991 CBCL/4-18, YSR, and TRF profiles.* Burlington, VT: University of Vermont Department of Psychiatry.

Deater-Deckard, K. (1996). *The Parent Feelings Questionnaire.* London: Institute of Psychiatry.

Goodman, R. (1997). The strengths and difficulties questionnaire: A research note. *Journal of Child Psychology and Psychiatry, 38,* 581-586.

McRoy, R.G., Zurcher, L.A., Lauderdale, M.L., and Anderson, R.N. (1982). Self esteem and racial identity in transracial and inracial adoptees. *Social Work, 27,* 522-526.

Rescorla, L., Hyson, M., Hirsch-Pasek, K., and Cone, J. (1990). Academic expectations in mothers of preschool children. *Early Education and Development, 1,* 165-184.

Schaefer, E. and Edgerton, M. D. (1985). Parent and child correlates of parental modernity. In I. Sigel (Ed.), *Parent belief systems: The psychological consequences for children,* First edition (pp. 287-318). Hillside, NJ: Erlbaum.

Tessler, R., Gamache, G., and Liu, L. (1996). *The bi-cultural Chinese American child socialization questionnaire.* Amherst, MA: University of Massachusetts.

U.S. Department of Education, National Center for Education Statistics (2001). Degrees and Other Formal Awards Conferred (survey); Integrated Postsecondary Education Data System (IPEDS), Completions (survey); and Earned Degrees Conferred Model.

Chapter 3

From Couple to Family

Naomi Moessinger

We are Naomi and Fred, aged sixty-seven and seventy-three, respectively, in 2002. We are both college graduates with no advanced degrees. We are a couple in which the wife is actively Jewish and the husband was born a Christian but practices no religion. Little did we realize that our intermarriage would become a huge impediment on our road to adoption in the United States. Fred was a vice president of Human Resources at Philip Morris International and did a lot of traveling all over the world. Perhaps his extensive traveling made the idea of international adoption not a big deal. I stayed home during the children's childhood and did a lot of volunteer work.

HOW WE GOT TO BE A FAMILY OF SEVENTEEN

We were married in late 1958 and decided by the spring of 1959 to stop using birth control so that we could conceive. I did conceive, several times, and then I would have very early miscarriages. I cannot remember how many times I miscarried, but I did go to the Margaret Sanger Clinic in New York City, which was considered the place to go for reproductive issues. We finished all the tests and they could find absolutely nothing wrong with either of us.

At that point we decided to adopt a child. Adoption had been discussed long before our marriage, and both of us were very comfortable with the idea. Our problem in trying to adopt was that we had an intermarriage, and that is where we got mired. We contacted Louise Wise, the Jewish adoption agency, which would not even interview us. We tried with the then-popular Caritas Agency, which was placing Greek babies in American homes, but I was not a Christian. At the time of our search, Greece was the main European country where there were children available for adoption. Greece in the early 1960s was still an extremely poor country. For example, much of the countryside was still without electricity, television had yet to be introduced, there was no social safety net in place, abortion was totally unavailable, and if a young woman unfortunately got pregnant, she needed to be able to find a family who would take care of her child.

If memory serves me correctly, the phrases "open adoption" or "closed adoption" were not used. At that time, however, I believe there was either a six- or twelve-month waiting period in New York State before an in-state adoption could become final. There were a few cases in the early 1960s of birth mothers changing their minds in that time period and the adoptive parents fleeing New York, usually to Florida. Most of the cases involved Jewish adoptive parents and a non-Jewish birth mother. The news articles convinced me that the only possible way I could be comfortable would be if the adoption that was totally fixed in stone legally.

We actually had very few options. No American agency would talk to us, as we were of different religions. I was scared to death of the concept of so-called black-market babies. A lawyer usually arranged adoption of a black-market baby, and the legality of the adoption tended not to be clear-cut. I simply could not deal with the fear—fear that every time the phone rang it could be the birth mother, or every time I went to open the mail, it could be a letter from a lawyer representing the birth mother. I also could not deal with the uncertainty of whose baby it was.

We were stuck, until a close friend who was a lawyer happened to mention a first cousin who lived next door to a couple in Merrick, Long Island (New York), who had just returned from Greece with an infant. When our friend found out that the couple was also Jewish, we became ecstatic, and on March 10, 1962, we drove to meet the couple and their new daughter. They gave us all the information that we needed to contact the lawyer in Greece, and we raced home and wrote a letter to the lawyer that very day (Fred's birthday). In the letter, I stated that I wanted a newborn infant. Fred immediately objected to that description and said that we should pick the sex. I looked at him and told him that I could not possibly play God and choose, so Fred chose an infant daughter. His reasoning was that he wanted me to have the same close relationship with a daughter that I had had with my mother.

On March 19, 1962, I opened the mailbox and out popped a letter with all sorts of strange stamps with very strange writing on them. It was a letter from the lawyer in Greece assuring us that we could definitely legally adopt a baby in Greece and he would be glad to handle the project himself. He also told us what his fees were ($1,500) and what documentation we needed to bring. He agreed to meet us at the airport and to take care of the hotel arrangements in Athens once we could give him definite dates and flight numbers. The list of required documents, as best we can recall, included a copy of our birth certificates, a copy of our marriage license, and notarized copies of our financial worth, whether it be in stocks, savings, real estate, or other forms. (The more financially comfortable we were, the better the chance of Greek judges approving us as suitable parents.) We also needed a letter of recommendation from an elected official. As for our suitability as parents, the home study by the U.S. government would be done while we were in Greece.

In retrospect, if we had been deemed unsuitable to become parents by the U.S. government, we would have been in deep trouble, as the Greek side of the adoption would have been concluded before we were ever declared fit parents. Thus, we would have ended up being parents, but parents without a country to go to. I do not remember that being a source of worry for us, as we knew not only that we were fit parents but also that we would be excellent parents. Getting the documents that the lawyer wanted so that we could proceed with the adoption was not difficult, other than getting a letter from an elected official. Living in the crowded area of Jackson Heights, Queens (New York), we knew no elected officials at all. Someone suggested that we immediately join the local Democratic Club (which we did) and then make a donation to the state senator of our district (which we did). Then we asked for a letter of recommendation stating that we were upstanding citizens and would also be good adoptive parents. The senator wrote what we needed him to say and we added the letter to our growing file. Since we wanted to show that we were as affluent as we could be, my mother transferred about $1,000 from her bank account to ours. As far as any psychologist, social worker, or government official getting involved with us before we left for Greece, there were none. We were on our own, with few or no guarantees that we would become parents, other than knowing that the couple in Merrick had succeeded in becoming parents to an infant. That is, it could be and had been done.

We arrived in Athens on May 1, 1962, and, as promised, our attorney met us at the airport. He told us that he had had difficulty getting us a hotel room, as there was a royal wedding about to take place and all the better hotels around were fully booked. He was rather embarrassed when he told us that he had booked us in a hotel in a not exactly wonderful area of the city called Omonia Square, but we would have to spend only about a week there, then the wedding guests would depart and we could move into an upscale hotel. The good thing about the hotel was that it was very inexpensive, but we did not care about the hotel at that time. We certainly did not expect to spend an extended amount of time in Athens. We had been told by the contact family in Merrick that we would be in Greece for only about two weeks.

In his car, the attorney told us that he was taking us to his apartment where he had ten infant girls waiting for us. I think that I must have asked him how old the youngest of the babies was, and I remember he said that she was born on April 20. From the backseat my husband announced that that day was Hitler's birthday. I gave him a scathing look. I also remember the lawyer asking us if we had anything in our respective backgrounds that could and would come out during an American background investigation. If so, he needed to know upfront so he would not receive any surprises. The only thing we could think of was the fact that in the 1930s my father may have been a member of the Communist Party. The lawyer did not think that would turn out to be an issue at all, as my father had then gone on to serve in the U.S. Marines during World War II and had earned an honorable discharge. We had never been arrested, and our only "run-in" with the law had been a ticket for not putting enough change in a parking meter. Fred had been drafted into the Army during the Korean War and had served as a cryptologist in the Counter Intelligence Corps.

Our attorney knew that we were intermarried, and he told us how he had taken care of this potential problem. Maurice, our attorney, was himself a Greek Jew who had married a Greek Christian. Maurice tended to wait to file adoption papers of an intermarried couple in the Court of First Instance in Athens until he knew who the three judges would be on any particular date. He also tried to get these cases heard very late in the day, at a time when most people, including judges, would like to go home. He was well aware of our intermarriage situation and had solved that problem by telling us that if a judge were to ask our religion, Fred, and only Fred, was to answer since technically he was a Christian. Therefore there would be no perjury in the courtroom. If, however, a judge were to ask me, then I would have to commit perjury, as no court in Greece would allow a Greek child to be adopted by a Jewish parent. He absolutely did not think that this would be a problem. I did not like the idea of committing perjury, but we had no other option.

By this time we had gotten to his apartment building, which was on a wide boulevard in a very posh neighborhood. We took the elevator upstairs and entered his apartment. What I remember is that the living room was furnished in a very traditional European look with dark wood furniture and heavy drapes. He excused himself, then came back with an infant swaddled in a flannel receiving blanket and placed her in my arms. I was overwhelmed that this tiny child could become my daughter. She was a little fussy, and Fred asked to hold her. Fred's magic began and she stopped fussing and gave him a crooked little smile. Maurice beamed and told us that there were nine other babies in another room just waiting for us. Again, I took my earlier stance and informed Maurice that I had no interest in "playing God" and thus had no interest at all in seeing another baby. This was our very own daughter and that is what mattered to me. Fred completely concurred. Maurice really tried to get us to look at the other infant girls, but we had no desire to see any others. Later on during our stay in Athens, we found out that we were the total exception. Most of the adoptive parents looked over every baby that Maurice was able to show them. We were also unaware that most American couples who traveled to Greece to adopt were much more interested in adopting boys, hence the surplus of infant girls. Fred gave our new daughter back to me and I held her again with a feeling of awe. It was then time to leave his apartment, get the ball rolling, and start all the paperwork that we needed to complete.

In the car, our lawyer again apologized for the hotel, which was in a seedy area of Athens. The hotel was very new and very, very plain, but it cost us only four dollars a night, including taxes and a continental breakfast. It was also very clean.

Maurice had arranged an appointment at the American Embassy, where we needed to have an interview, our baby needed a physical,

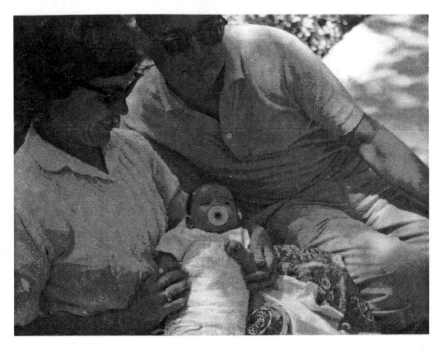

Naomi and Fred with Deborah, May 1962

and, of course, we needed to fill out all sorts of forms so we could start the home review process in the United States. Our daughter's name was to be Deborah Joy. She was cared for by a woman and her family in the port city of Athens, called Piraeus. The nanny met us at the embassy late in the morning. Deborah was presented to us swaddled in a pink-and-blue wool blanket. She was peacefully sleeping. It was May 2, and she was all of twelve days old. We sat on a wooden bench awaiting our interview with Vice Consul Hawthorne Mills. As we nervously waited, an American woman passed by and peered down at the sleeping infant. She looked at the infant and proud mother and pronounced the baby beautiful. Then, to cap it off, she told us that the baby looked just like me! The interview with the ambassador's assistant was short and unmemorable. We filled out forms that had to be sent to the United States for the home study and to the FBI and the New York Police Department.

Next we met the embassy doctor, who unwrapped Deborah and did a very perfunctory checkup. He told us that she needed to have a phenylketonuria (PKU) test as soon as we got back to the states. He listened to her heart, looked in her eyes and ears, weighed her and measured her, and that was that. Back in the United States I had visited the pediatrician whom I planned to use and had asked him what medical questions I should ask. In 1962, there was very little testing that could be done. He suggested that she be checked for tuberculosis (TB). The embassy doctor did the TB test. As soon as the interview and medical checkup were done, Deborah was whisked away by her nanny. The nanny did not speak a word of English, and we did not speak a word of Greek. (The only Greek I could read was capital letters that represented fraternities.)

The rest of the week we spent sightseeing in Athens, as our court date was not until May 7. Maurice anticipated that after the court date, if all went smoothly, we would have Deborah's American visa within two weeks. Rather than spend the two weeks in Athens, we decided that we should do some sightseeing, as we might never have the chance again. We took a bus to Piraeus and looked at the dates and prices for a tour of the Greek Islands. We found a boat that met our requirements (i.e., it was inexpensive). For seventy dollars a person we could go on a five-day cruise with everything included. The departure date was good, as the boat left a few days after the court hearing. So we booked the cruise, which departed from Piraeus on May 14.

By Monday, May 7 (the day of the adoption proceedings), we were nervous. Would everything go right? Would I have to perjure myself? Fred and I dressed in the fashion of the day: suit, white shirt, and tie for Fred, and dress, stockings, and heels for me. Maurice's legal assistant picked us up and took us to the courthouse. It was about 7 p.m., and the court and the courtroom were surprisingly empty. We were ushered into the courtroom, where three judges in black robes were sitting at a long table. I looked around the courtroom and noticed a woman sitting alone who, in my eyes, looked exactly like a prostitute. She was dressed in a very tight sapphire blue dress and shoes. I remember thinking that I did not want her to be the birth mother, although I knew that the birth mother would be in the courtroom. Obviously all the speaking was done in Greek, and our attorney was up at the table talking to the judges of the Court of First Instance. The only question they asked Fred was how much money he made. He answered in English ($11,000), and it was translated into Greek drachmas. There was a gasp from the few spectators in the room. Obviously, we were considered affluent and whatever faults we might have disappeared with Fred's answer. In a few more minutes the hearing was over and we were declared (in Greek, of course) the parents of the illegitimate, unbaptized child of Anastasia Argyrous, daughter of Alexander Argyrous. It was over and we were now parents. It was so anticlimactic.

AND WE WAIT AND WAIT AND WAIT . . .

Maurice came over to congratulate us and then led us out of the courtroom. He told us that there was someone he wanted us to meet. He introduced us to the birth mother, Anastasia, and her aunt and uncle. Anastasia's hometown was on the island of Corfu (an island off the west coast of Greece), and, not unlike many other women, when she became pregnant, she left Corfu and came to Athens to stay with her aunt and uncle until she gave birth. In 1962, in conservative Greece, an out-of-wedlock birth was cause for great shame. During the time that we were in Athens, there was a story in the English-language newspaper about a woman who gave birth to an illegitimate child and refused to give up the child for adoption, and how basically she was homeless and had no money for food or shelter. In the Greece of 1962, there was absolutely no safety net at all.

Maurice had neglected to tell me that I would have to meet the birth mother. Since she and her family spoke no English and we spoke no Greek, Maurice had to interpret for us. No, Anastasia was not the woman who looked like a hooker. My memory of her was that she was even shorter than I am and was very young and frightened-looking. Tradition had it that we should have gone out to a café for coffee and cake, but I told Maurice I simply could not do this. Anastasia touched my arm, and that was that. We were now the parents of an eighteen-day-old beautiful daughter. Now all we had to do was to collect her visa from the American Embassy and fly home.

The next day, Maurice's legal assistant, Marina, picked us up, as we had to go to some Greek administrative building to fill out forms for Deborah's Greek passport, for translations of the adoption hearing into English, and for the issuance of a birth certificate. These forms then had to be submitted to the American Embassy. We walked into a building, and Marina found the counter she was looking for and plunged into a large group of people, all pushing and shoving to get to the counter and get the attention of one of the clerks. The scene was one of total chaos. Calmly, Marina pushed and shoved us to the front of the desk, put down the filled-out forms, gave the clerk some drachmas, and was given some receipts in return. The clerks were very busy, using lots of stamps to mark the receipts. This procedure was followed two more times at two more counters on different floors. I vividly remember thinking that if we had had to do this on our own, we would have never gotten past the first counter. All the writing in the building was in Greek, and in 1962 very few people spoke English at all. Finally, I thought we were done, but Marina said we had one more set of papers that had to be stamped by the head of the Passport Division in order for Deborah's Greek passport to be issued.

We were ushered into a very large and spacious office. After the cramped and dirty counters and the shoving and pushing, this was an oasis. An air of calm prevailed. At the big desk sat the man who was going to put on the final stamps we needed to get the passport. He graciously asked us to sit down on the other side of his desk. I noticed right away that he had ice blue eyes. I thought of the Gestapo. He was very courteous to us as he glanced over the papers that Marina had set in front of him. He made a few inconsequential comments, and then he asked if the name Deborah was a Jewish name. Marina was struck dumb by the question, and even Fred, who is usually quick to answer, just sat there. I told him that I did not know if it was a Jewish name or not, but that it was a very popular name back home in the United States. I then dropped the names of Debbie Reynolds and Deborah Kerr, explaining that Debbie was the nickname of Deborah. He fixed his steely blue eyes on mine and we locked eyes. I did not flinch. Then he wanted to know why we had not had the baby baptized. I never moved my eyes from him as I explained that we were planning to have the baby baptized at home so that all our family and friends could celebrate. However, if he wanted us to we would be delighted to have a baptism in Athens. He would have to help us arrange it and we would be delighted if he would be the godfather. There was complete silence in the room. I doubt if the silence lasted more than ten seconds, but to the three of us it seemed an eternity. I never blinked but just calmly sat there staring at him, and after the eternity had passed, he picked up the stamps that were needed to issue Deborah a passport. We picked up the papers, said thank you, and left. Fred and Marina looked at me. They had been stunned into silence with his question about our daughter's name. Fortunately, from somewhere deep inside me came the calm and glibness needed so that he would stamp the required documents. Later that day, Maurice apologized profusely. It turned out that the man had been newly appointed to his position, and now Maurice knew that it was going to be difficult to deal with him on matters of religion until some money changed hands.

Two days later we left on the TSS *Aegean* for our five-day cruise of the Greek islands. In 1962, Greece was not yet much of a tourist destination, so we spent five wonderful days in May without the hassle of other tourists. We came back to Athens excited by what we had seen and experienced and ready to hear some positive news from Maurice about the status of our obtaining Deborah's American visa. There was no news at all and we were disappointed, but he explained that it was much too early. We spent Sunday at Maurice's beach house in Vouligmeni, where we met a lovely American couple who had just arrived. They were planning to adopt an infant boy. We hit it off and spent a lot of time with them. By the middle of the following week, we still had no answer. We went to the embassy more than once, and each time we walked away very disappointed. We did manage to see Deborah once or twice, and then we decided to go to Israel. The plane fare was not much, and my parents had friends in Tel Aviv who immediately invited us to stay with them. We flew to Israel and landed the night before the fourteenth anniversary of the birth of Israel. We were in Israel for about one week and managed to see many wonderful sights, but our hearts were really back in Athens.

The day we got back to Athens we immediately called Maurice, who still had no information for us. He invited us over to his apartment for dinner. After a lovely dinner, during the course of which I became more and more nauseated, I ended up being very sick to my stomach. The next night I also vomited and thought that I had caught a virus. The weather was turning hot, and our small hotel had no air-conditioning at all. We were both becoming very depressed. We spent some more time with Deborah, but Fred was seriously considering leaving and going back to the United States to return to work. He would leave me to bring Deborah home. The days went slowly; I felt sick, and the heat was intense. We certainly had no money to go to a first-class hotel with air-conditioning. We took a trip to Delphi and did some shopping, but we were both becoming very concerned about Deborah's visa.

THE TRANSATLANTIC PHONE CALL

We spent hours trying to figure out what could have gone wrong. The American Embassy would telex the Department of Immigration and Naturalization, but we never got an answer as to what was happening. Finally, the couple whom we had met at Maurice's beach house offered to help us. His brother worked for the American Embassy in Rome, so he called his brother for us. His brother suggested that we call the head of the Eastern Division of Immigration and Naturalization. In 1962, it was not easy to place an international phone call. You called the international operator and gave her the phone number you wanted to reach. The operator would take the information and then tell you about how long it would take to put the call through. It could take hours.

We went back to our room and Fred placed the call. It was Thursday, June 7, and because of the time difference, although it was late in the afternoon in Athens, it was morning in New York. Finally the operator called us back. I heard Fred ask for Mr. Esterhazy (the head of the Eastern Division of Immigration and Naturalization). Fred then gave his name, adding that he was an American citizen. Fred spoke to Mr. Esterhazy for a few minutes, telling him our tale of woe. I heard a few "Hahums," "OK," and then a "Thank you very much." He hung up the phone and turned to me. Mr. Esterhazy had promised him an answer the next day. The rest of the day dragged by. By then Athens had turned unbearably hot. The hotel had given us a tiny, tiny fan. The streets were filled with diesel fumes and I was incredibly nauseous.

June 8 dawned, and again we had to wait until the afternoon to reach New York because of the time difference. This time the call to New York did not take as long. I was stretched out on the bed in our tiny room, holding the hand fan, when the operator rang. Fred picked up the phone, listened, and said something like, "Thank you very much." He hung up the phone, turned to me, and said, "It's all over." I burst out crying because I interpreted those words to mean "no Deborah." He was equally stunned because he knew that the words meant that the wait was over and we could take our daughter and fly home. We had a million errands to do that afternoon, so we separated. Fred ran to the American Embassy to pick up her visa, and I ran to the airlines to put us on the Saturday, June 9, flight. Although we had flown over on Icelandic Air (to save money), we realized that we could not do that returning because of the length of the trip. In our free time wandering around Athens, we had decided to use SwissAir. They were most accommodating because they offered to have diapers in Zurich, where we were due to have a stopover. We had dinner with Maurice and his wife and some other friends. Then, as usual, at 11:00 p.m. I vomited and then went on with my life.

WE GET TO GO HOME

Our new life as parents actually began on the morning of June 9 as the nanny brought Deborah to me with a blue-and-pink wool blanket, an outfit that we had bought, a pacifier, and two bottles with formula. There was also a container with more formula. We had one diaper, and Deborah was swaddled. (Diapers were unavailable in Greece at that time as all Greeks swaddled infants.) Of course, in 1962 disposable diapers had not come on the market even in the United States. We had also bought a baby carrier that airlines (at that time) recommended. We taxied to the airport and were there at about 6 a.m. After checking through the tickets, passports, visas, etc., we were finally in the departure lounge. The hotel dining room had not been open when we checked out, so Fred left me to get some breakfast. For the first time I was on my own. By then Deborah was screaming in her carrier, so I picked her up and tried to give her a bottle, but she would not stop screaming. In desperation I put her back down on her back, but she was still screaming and spitting out her pacifier. An English grandmotherly type approached me, looked into the carrier, and said very gently, "Why don't you try putting the baby on her stomach." I did and in one minute she was fast asleep!

We eventually boarded the plane for Zurich. I was anxious to be given some diapers because I was very aware that we were skating on thin ice without them. Unfortunately for us, the airport in Zurich was closed down due to bad weather, and we had to refuel in Geneva, where there were no diapers for us. I kept refolding the giant diaper as needed. After Geneva, we had to make a stop in Lisbon for refueling and cleaning the aircraft before we left to cross the Atlantic. SwissAir let Deborah and me stay on the flight, as she was sound asleep and I just did not want to move her again. The Portuguese cleaners oohed and aahed over our fifty-day-old infant. Finally we were flying over the Atlantic. Every time I needed to heat a bottle, they stopped serving in the kitchen and Deborah got first priority. Somewhere over the Atlantic, the crew, including the pilot and copilot, presented us with a book of Swiss fairy tales in English, and every employee on the flight signed it, along with a notation that it was her very first flight. The flight was rather unremarkable because Deborah woke to eat, fussed, and then slept for an hour or two. We landed at Idlewild (now JFK) airport late in the afternoon. We were beyond exhausted. As we went through immigration we had one testy moment. The immigration agent looking over Deborah's papers and visa announced to me that she was not vaccinated and therefore would have to be quarantined for fourteen days. I stared at him with a vacant look and then handed Deborah to him. I told him that either he would have to believe that I had a pediatrician's appointment for the coming Monday or he could personally keep her and we would pick her up after fourteen days. I am not sure if I was playing chicken or not. All I remember of that moment was that I was incredibly exhausted and I just wanted to be left alone. We glared at each other for some seconds, and then he picked up the stamp and let her in. Welcome to America!

We went into the baggage area to wait for our luggage. In those days, there was a glass wall separating the passengers from those waiting to pick them up. We picked out my mom, Fred's parents, and my very close friends, Bernice and Allan, and their two young sons. They were waving a pink dog at us. A few minutes later, as we were gazing at the carousel waiting for our bags, someone grabbed me from the back and said, "Give me Deborah." It was my mother. She had talked to the police at the door and told them that she had waited seven weeks for this day and could not wait another second, and they let her enter the baggage claim area, which of course is before you clear customs. I remember being amazed that she had managed to come into the baggage area. We made our way through customs with my mother holding fiercely onto Deborah, and then once we were out in the pickup area, Fred's parents and Bernice and Allan and their kids began oohing and aahing over our new daughter. We were driven home to our apartment building.

At 6 p.m., I gave Deborah a bottle and put her down in her brand-new crib, and she fell right asleep. Fred was smart. He got into bed and fell asleep. I could not, because every neighbor wanted to see Deborah. It was a long evening of people pouring in to wish us congratulations, and as I crawled into bed at midnight, Deborah woke up.

She thought it was 6 a.m. and she needed to eat, but she also was wide-awake! Oh well, welcome to motherhood. Obviously the only real adjustment problem was the profound time change, which I managed by moving her clock around in fifteen-minute intervals.

Fred called Mr. Esterhazy to find out what had taken so long. The answer was that they were moving the New York City Police Department files, and the files that started with the letter "M" had been sealed and were not due to be unsealed anytime in the future. He, of course, had managed to have them unsealed, and of course our names were not in the files.

WE VERY QUICKLY BECOME A FAMILY OF FIVE

On January 13, 1963, eight months and three weeks after Deborah's birth, I gave birth to a wonderful baby boy named Mark. All that vomiting had been because I was pregnant. Only after Mark was born and I had another infant to compare her to did it dawn on me that Deborah really did not recognize me as her mom (caretaker) for quite a while. On January 8, 1968, I gave birth to an infant girl we named Sarah. From the moment Sarah came home, Deborah, who was not quite six, became her "other mother," caretaker, and good friend.

Even before we actually had Deborah, Fred and I had known that she would not grow up being told that she was a birth child. There was literally no literature out there for adopted children other than a book called *The Chosen Baby* (now out of print).

Our children were rather attached to one another. Deborah and Sarah were, and still are, very close. One lives in New Jersey and the other in Wisconsin, and they talk on the phone to each other many times a week. In the early years, Mark was more allied to Deborah, as they were so close in age. When they were very young, an Irish friend of mine told me that they were what the Irish call "Irish twins" because they were born within a year of each other but were not actually twins. They were natural playmates and managed to engage in lots of mischief, as they each had the other to feed off of.

In the spring of 1973, Fred had to make a business trip to Europe, and we decided that I would take both Deborah and Mark to Greece and meet Fred in Athens. We did this over the children's spring break from school and spent two wonderful weeks in Greece, seeing Athens and the Pelopenessian Peninsula and making the obligatory tour of the Greek Islands. That one trip to Greece was about as much as we did to educate Deborah in her birth heritage. Deborah has also not shown much interest in the fact that she is Greek. I hope that someday she and her husband will visit Greece.

Living in suburban New Jersey at a time when you could let your children roam free in the neighborhood, Deborah grew up knowing that she was adopted. We had never made a big deal about it, and although neighbors knew, it just was not an issue. She and her brother never realized how odd it was that she was only nine months older than he was. She tells me that they never had a discussion about the fact that they were so close in age. In fact, she does not remember Mark ever discussing with her the fact that she was adopted, even though, as close as they were, they tended to share their feelings and their thoughts with each other. Neither Sarah nor Mark has ever asked us if we loved Deborah any differently than we loved them. She was our eldest daughter and child. To us, it was just that simple.

Deborah has our coloring, and I remember once at a fifth-grade conference the teacher remarked as I walked into the room that she would have picked me out as being Deborah's mother because we looked so much alike. However, when Deborah was in high school and beyond we had many problems. There was even a year that we were not in contact with each other. Was it due to adoption? Now that Deborah is fast approaching her fortieth birthday and we are wonderfully close, she still cannot give either herself or us an answer.

The one difference that we could ever see between two birth children and an adopted child was that both our birth children and their parents are incredible readers. We all love to read. Deborah, to this day, is not much of a reader. On the other hand, a year ago Sarah went shopping, in Milwaukee, for a dress to wear to a bat mitzvah. Deborah also went shopping, in New Jersey, for a dress to wear to the same bat mitzvah. Were they ever surprised when they realized they had both bought the same dress.

Even if I had been given a look into the future at all the pitfalls we would encounter with Deborah in her teen years, I definitely would repeat the experience and have always suggested adoption to couples who cannot have children on their own.

Life is a journey, and Deborah started us on the road to the wonderful experience of being parents and grandparents. Deborah, Mark, and Sarah each have married. Deborah is the mother of four children,

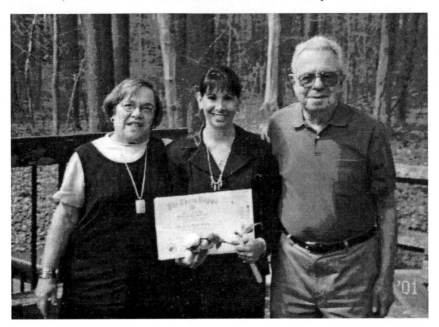

Naomi, Deborah, and Fred

Mark of three, and Sarah of two. We are the very proud grandparents of five grandsons and four granddaughters ranging in age from one year to twenty-one years. Oh, yes, Deborah still has the forty-year-old, worn-out stuffed pink poodle that her Aunt Bernice and Uncle Allan gave her on June 9, 1962.

ADDENDUM BY DEBORAH JOHNSON

Everyone loves to hear their parents tell the story of the day they were born. This is true for me, too, although my story differs a lot from those of other people. I used to ask my parents to tell me the story over and over again because I loved to hear it.

The story began in Athens, Greece. I would always ask my dad to tell me what happened the first time he saw me. I was very curious to know how I was chosen. My parents always said that they could have had many choices of babies while in Greece. They were offered twins, but they were not interested in twins. They were also offered

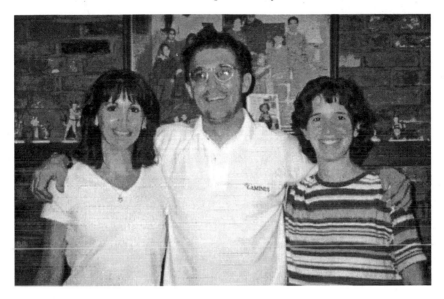

Deborah, Mark, and Sarah, July 1999

the chance to look at many babies and pick the one they wanted. My mother always said that would have been too hard a choice, that she would feel like she was playing God.

My parents were taken to the lawyer's home, where many babies were waiting to be adopted. My parents had told the lawyer ahead of time that they wanted an infant girl. They agreed that they would take the first baby he brought out. I was the first baby. The story goes on that as my dad held me for the first time, I smiled at him. That is the story of my birth as far as I am concerned.

My birth story continues at Kennedy Airport where my mom, my dad, and I were just coming in from Athens. My mom usually told this story. She would laugh as she told how her mother, my "mama," found her way through customs, which was always off limits to anyone other than the people exiting or entering the airplane. She told the airport security guard that she had waited long enough to see her grandchild and would not wait another minute. From that day till her death, my mama and I had a very special relationship.

Two other people present at my arrival were my parents' best friends, my Aunt Bernice and Uncle Allan. They waited for me with a gift, a pink stuffed puppy. I grew up with that puppy and took it everywhere I went throughout my childhood. It sits in my room to this day and brings back wonderful memories of my arrival in the United States. In July 2002, my Uncle Allan passed away. Because he was very special to me from my arrival in the United States until his death, I would like to dedicate my story to him. He will be missed.

I never thought it was out of the ordinary that I was adopted. I never thought it was odd that my brother, Mark, and I were so close in age. It never struck me as odd that for three months out of the year we were actually the same age. I was always happy to have a sibling so close in age to play with. We were not in the same grade in school, though, so I always thought of myself as the older sister.

We never talked about the fact that I was adopted unless I asked to hear a story about it. I always knew I was adopted. I never had to have my parents sit down and tell me that I was an adopted child because they were always so open about telling the birth story. I always knew.

I was from Greece, so my appearance did not bring up any adoption questions from other people. I had brown hair and brown eyes just like everyone else in my family. Sometimes, I would not think about the fact that I was adopted for years. I just grew up. My brother never talked about it and, of course, never treated me differently. He treated me just like any brother would treat a sister. When my younger sister was born six years later, I was in heaven. I had a sister to take care of. I do not even know how my brother and sister found out about the fact that I was adopted. We all just fit like such a great family that it was never really an issue.

All of my friends knew that I was adopted. I always told everyone I was born in Greece. I was proud of the fact that I was chosen. I always thought it was so great to come from another country. No one I knew ever reacted in a negative way about the fact that I was adopted, so I always had a great experience with it. Maybe it would have been different all those years ago if I had come from a country where my appearance was different from the rest of my family. Who knows?

When I was in fourth grade, my family and I visited Greece. We had a foster child, Peter, over there, whom my parents had been sponsoring for years, and this gave us the opportunity to meet him. I also got the opportunity to see the country where I was born. Although we did not actually visit the island my birth mother had come from, Corfu, we saw many other islands, and I got a real taste of my heritage. I enjoyed that trip more than any other we would take in later years. I have not been back to Greece since, but I would love to visit again with my family to show my children where I came from.

My life went on like any child's until my teenage years. I got a little lost at that time, as many teenagers do, and ended up having my first child at age eighteen years. For some reason, this triggered a need in me to search for my birth mother. I do not know if it was a natural reaction because I had just had a child, or if maybe I needed to search because my relationship with my own parents had become nonexistent at that point because of the choices I had made for myself.

I had no idea where to start. I was living in Pennsylvania at the time, and there were no resources like the Internet in 1980. I decided to call the United Nations in New York. A very kind man there sent me the phone book directory for the island of Corfu. I knew my birth mother's name and decided to start there. I composed a letter and brought it to a Greek Orthodox Church where a kind priest translated it into Greek for me. I mailed a copy to every Argyrous in the phone book. That would be the equivalent of mailing a letter to every Smith in an American phone book. Next, I contacted the New York office of the lawyer who had handled the adoption and wrote a letter to him. At that point in time it was all I could do. I never had a response from anyone.

As the years went on and my relationship with my parents started to heal, I lost interest in searching. Frankly, it was very time-consuming and I did not have the time to put into it. My interest was sparked again when I read a *People* magazine in 1996 with an article in it about illegal adoptions out of Greece dated to the 1950s and early 1960s. As I read the article, to my horror I discovered that the lawyer who was stealing these babies from their mothers and shipping them to the United States was the same lawyer who had handled my adoption. My search began again at this point.

I found out that you could write to INS (Immigration and Naturalization Services), and they would send you your INS file. That was my first step. It took about five months to get my file. In the meantime, I had found an online mailing list for Greek adoptees on the Internet and joined it. Through these e-mails I learned of Litsa, a woman in Florida who would search for Greek adoptees' birth parents. Her fee was minimal, $125. The only stipulation was that if she found family members she would give out only your information. If they did not want to be contacted she would not give you their information.

A couple of months later I got the call that Litsa had found my birth mother. She said she was interested in contacting me. I found out that she had been living in Astoria, Queens, for years. I was so excited, and my mom and dad, who had been totally supportive of the search, were excited, too. I was in contact with her and her family by phone for a while, although it was hard because my birth mother did not really speak English. Finally, they mailed me a picture of their family. That was the day it hit me—hard. This was not my family. My family was right in Holmdel, New Jersey, where they had always been. I lost interest in having any contact with my birth mother. I realized that I had no feelings for this woman, except gratitude for giving me up for adoption and enabling me to have a wonderful life.

Through the years I had developed such a close relationship with my parents that I have no need to connect with my birth mother. The old saying "Be careful what you wish for" is the saying I live by now. I wished to find my birth mother, and when I found her I realized that I had never really wanted to meet her. I share this story with my own four children and hope they learn from it. I am glad I have some information about my birthplace to share with my children.

Not all adoptees have such a happy life with their adopted families. The key to our family is that we never acted like I was different, because I was not. Your family is who raises you, cares for you when you are sick, goes through the good and the bad with you while still loving you no matter what. Anyone can have a baby; not everyone can be a parent. I was lucky to have been chosen by a couple who really wanted to be parents and who devoted their lives to me, my brother, and my sister to build an unbreakable relationship, which we continue to have to this day.

Chapter 4

Coming Home from China

Margaret V. Moro

THE POTENTIAL PARENTS

At forty-four years of age, I got married for the first time to a divorced, childless man who was six years my junior. A year and a half later, Joel and I attended the wedding of one of my colleagues and were seated next to a couple. In conversation, they told us that they were waiting to adopt a baby girl from China. They were expecting to receive news from the adoption agency at any time, advising them to travel to China.

My initial reaction was disbelief. She was forty-six years of age, he was forty-three; this was her second marriage and his first; they were married only a few years longer than we; and they were both psychotherapists. I felt a great deal of identification with their life cycle and free-spirited lifestyle but could not understand why they would want to ruin their lives at this point with child rearing. I was a marriage and family therapist and knew indirectly about child rearing. It required a commitment to the child, a loss of personal freedom, and a certain amount of sacrifice.

I asked why they were going to adopt. With patience they answered this and my many other questions about adoption in China. I did not know about China's one-child policy or about the historical abandonment of female babies there because of the Chinese belief in the superior worth of male babies. China's social structure leaves the obligation of care for elderly parents to the sons and their wives. Tradition holds that when the females marry, they leave their families to live with and care for their husbands' families. This means parents of females have no one to care for them in their later years, and the government does not offer any assistance, so all parents want sons.

Our Reasons for Adopting

There is an old Chinese saying that females are like grass to be stepped on. When I realized that little girls were being thrown away because of their sex, I felt pangs of empathy. I had experienced gender discrimination in my own family of origin as the only daughter with three older brothers. I was drawn to the women's movement in the 1970s because of this background and other family experiences, and I learned to value myself as a female. At some point during the aforementioned conversation, it became obvious to me that adopting a baby girl from China would fit right into my value system.

That evening in 1995, I learned about the eligibility requirements for adopting a healthy child from China. A couple had to have no children in their present marriage, be between thirty-five and sixty years old, and have at least $15,000 available to spend on the adoption. Single parents could also adopt. Finally, I learned of the existence of an organization called Families with Children from China (FCC) that was comprised of mostly Caucasian, middle-aged, middle-class professionals who had adopted babies from China. It was not anticipated then that, by 1999, China would change its adoption laws, drop the age requirements to thirty years old, and allow families to adopt a second child.

I left the wedding thinking, "I could do this." Finally, when I was forty-six years old, all the necessary elements were in place for me to become a parent. I was happily married and I knew that my husband would be ecstatic at the idea of adopting and parenting. This was my last opportunity for parenting, and I decided to take it!

In discussing our future together prior to our marriage, Joel and I accepted that the chances of a healthy baby coming from my body were not in our favor. We made the decision not to prevent or pursue pregnancy. We left the child issue up to Fate. We met Fate at the wedding when we began our consideration to adopt a Chinese baby girl.

OUR EXPERIENCES EN ROUTE TO THE ADOPTION

I called the adoption agency used by the couple we met at the wedding, and within a month Joel and I attended a lecture on international adoption. We learned that China had first opened its doors to international adoption in 1991 and that the process was still not smooth, but ultimately reliable. We would be guaranteed a healthy baby girl, but the process toward that end was unpredictable and inefficient by our standards. Chinese authorities wanted to ensure that those who raised their children were both financially stable and child centered. We looked no further.

We announced our intention to adopt at Christmas, and our families' responses were positive. Our baby would have a family with one grandparent in Colorado and a larger family with many second cousins near her age who lived in New Jersey. Her first cousins were of childbearing age.

We next had to fill out a tremendous amount of paperwork. First, we had to fill out a form for the Immigration and Naturalization Service (INS) so we could bring home an orphan from a foreign country. Our daughter would have her green card at the time of her arrival in the United States, and we would (and did) have to apply for citizenship for her at a later time. It took the INS three months to process our packet and return the necessary documentation. Prior to submitting this information, we had to get fingerprinted for a criminal background check. The Chinese government required copies of our birth certificates, our marriage certificate and Joel's divorce papers, and bank statements that showed $15,000 in our names. These all had to be certified, notarized, authenticated, and translated. We had to have a home study done by a licensed social worker. We reviewed our upbringing and reasons for adopting with the social worker, who then wrote a report recommending us as fit parents. This report, too, had to be translated. Finally, we had to include pictures of our home that clearly depicted the baby's room and a bathroom with a toilet. Since we had yet to set up our baby's room, I sent a picture of my niece's baby's room.

While going through this process, Joel and I began to notice other Caucasian parents with Chinese babies, and we immediately struck up conversations with them. Mostly the reaction from the parents was positive, and we learned from their experiences. An entire new world had begun to open up to us. The adoption agency hosted events during which returning and waiting families could socialize and interact. It was at one of these events that we again saw the couple we had met at the wedding, Timothy and Candice, with their daughter, Melody Joy Kwan Yin, a tiny baby, nine months old.

We had the feeling of belonging to a larger movement, since Chinese adoptions were gaining in popularity. Biracial families consisting of Chinese daughters and Caucasian parents were increasing annually because of the number of healthy girls available. Being a biracial family and an adoptive family was new to us, but we were not alone. There were others who walked ahead of us and with us. We knew that we, and especially our future daughter, would be the targets of prejudice, and, to the best of our abilities, we could prepare ourselves from others' experiences. Common stereotypes are that Asian women are exotic, the babies are beautiful, and the entire Asian population is smart. I wonder if it is better to have a positive stereotype than a negative one.

Finally, our agency sent the completed packet to China at the end of June 1996. Unbeknownst to us, June was the month our daughter was born and brought to the orphanage. It was also the month that we moved to a new home to be closer to my family. We were told we would probably travel to China in September. In September, we hosted a party for our adoption agency that included prospective adoptive parents, waiting parents, and families who had returned from China. We were told that we would not be going to China as expected because the government had closed the departments that governed the adoptions and were reorganizing. No one knew when applications would begin being processed again.

Although we were reassured that there was a healthy baby for us, I experienced periods of doubt and mistrust of the Chinese government during the waiting period. As I awoke to the news on the radio daily, I would listen intently to the news about China. Relations between the United States and China seemed tenuous at best. The more I read and learned, the more mistrusting of the People's Republic of China I became. This Communist government seemed to follow its own rules, which appeared to be very different from our democratic rules. I felt very powerless during the waiting time. My worst fear was that China would cut off relations with the United States.

Our wait continued. September turned to October, October turned to November, and still no word. By Thanksgiving, we were discouraged and frustrated. We knew that the Chinese government would be closed for two weeks from the end of January through sometime in February for the Chinese New Year. During this waiting time, I was completing my dissertation, and I wanted to finish it before I went to

China because I was not sure if I would be able to complete it with the responsibilities of motherhood. In many ways, working on the dissertation helped distract me from the adoption frustrations and parenting anticipations. I was successful in the defense of my dissertation in December 1996.

Around the same time, I received an invitation to travel to China with the People to People Ambassador Program. It was a tour for marriage and family therapists and psychologists from the United States to meet our Chinese counterparts. I knew psychotherapy per se was not available in China, but the tour would give me time in China to learn about the culture, as well as to meet interesting people. This would be my last time to travel alone. Since the trip was scheduled for March, I decided that I would take this trip, and I would want to pick up my baby while I was in China. With the dissertation completed I was ready to be a parent and was tired of waiting and feeling powerless. I discussed this plan with our adoption agency. I was told it might be possible since I would already be in China, and that because "Dr. Moro" was already in the country, the officials might respond favorably.

I signed up for the tour, anticipating that I would meet my husband after two weeks and we would go to get our daughter. And it did indeed happen this way. The agency notified the Chinese government that I would be in China, and the wheels were set in motion. I already had my traveling papers and visa.

Finally, we got the call from the agency in February that our referral had arrived. We were so excited, and now we would finally see a picture of our daughter. It was becoming real at last. Joel and I playfully argued over who was going to take the picture to work the next day.

When we saw the photo of our daughter-to-be, she looked like a three-month-old baby. We were given her date of birth (June 9, 1996) and the name of the town and province where she lived. Everything else was written in Chinese. She had no hair, big ears, and two little eyes that seemed to be looking right at us. We knew not to get attached to this child because, although this was the child they had selected for us, we might not end up with her as our daughter. We heard that occasionally a child got sick or died before the new parents arrived. Also, we were told that we had the option of refusing the child handed to us for whatever reason. In the event that we refused the child that they brought us, we were told that they would select another child. "Like a puppy pound," my brother said.

We made our travel arrangements with the adoption agency. I was scheduled to meet Joel on April 10 in Shanghai after my trip. We would then travel to Guangzhou, stay at the White Swan Hotel, a beautiful modern hotel very close to the American Consulate, and then we would travel to the town where our future daughter lived. The agency and others who had gone before us gave us a list of what to bring. We were ready. I left New York for China on Good Friday, March 28, 1997.

While waiting to board, I noticed that I was one of three Caucasians going to China on a packed airplane. When the announcement came to board the airplane, everyone rushed the gate. No one lined up to board the plane. Personal space seemed different for Chinese than for Americans. This observation would be consistent throughout our trip. The beginning of my introduction to Chinese culture had begun.

To read while traveling twenty-four hours, extended over a day and a half, I selected the book *China Wakes,* by Kristof and Wudunn (1994), two *New York Times* journalists. They described China since the "liberation" in 1949 when Chairman Mao closed China from the rest of the world. I was horrified and felt like I needed to hide this book. I thought that the Chinese officials would be angry and confiscate it if they knew what was written in it. I read about the repression and record of human rights violations, and this frightened me. I recalled that during my hippie days in the 1970s, Mao was held up as a hero. Now I was reading about the real Cultural Revolution, and not about some imagined folk hero version of what happened in China under his leadership. I began to feel very uncomfortable.

When I arrived in Beijing, a Chinese man who spoke English met me at the airport to drive me to the hotel where I would join the others on the People to People tour. It was Easter Sunday afternoon. The hotel was a modern high-rise with elevators and marble floors. The People to People information had said we would be staying in four- and five-star hotels. The major difference between U.S. and Chinese hotels was that in China women are stationed in each hallway, twenty-four hours a day, to distribute boiled water in thermoses for the guests to drink because the regular water is not drinkable.

On the tour we visited Beijing, Nanjing, Suzhou, and Shanghai, as well as the Great Wall. We listened to our Chinese colleagues talk about social conditions in China. We met the people who worked with social issues, those who did research, and those who made policy. They said there was no AIDS problem in China and there was no prostitution. They were concerned with the increase in divorce and violence and wanted to seek possible solutions. We ate some meals with them and spoke through translators.

There were no therapists as we know them in China, since Chinese Communism does not allow for personal freedoms such as free speech. I knew they were not telling us the whole truth; saving face, a phrase used to avoid humiliation and embarrassment, was an important value to them. We had to show respect to our hosts. Therefore, we could not discuss Tiananmen Square or talk about how and why they implemented the one-child policy. We could not discuss the fact that they were allowing their abandoned daughters to leave their country. There was so much I wanted to know.

My colleagues knew why I was in China: I was experiencing the country and culture of my soon-to-be daughter. Interestingly, our bilingual tour guides were perplexed. They did not know that China was allowing foreigners to adopt their children. They were curious as to why I wanted a little girl from China. After I explained that I was too old to have my own children, they seemed to understand. They all said how lucky she was.

Finally, I said good-bye to my colleagues after a wonderful send-off. Being with this group was the right thing for me. I felt nurtured and cared for by the many women there. The importance of my professional life seemed to be dwindling. I met Joel at 8 a.m. in the Shanghai Airport and we boarded a plane for Guangzhou.

In planning our travel arrangements, our adoption agency arranged for a Chinese guide for us. We were told that we needed a guide because it would be near impossible to negotiate China on our own, due to the language barrier and cultural differences. Peter, our guide, met us at the Guangzhou airport and took us to the White Swan Hotel, where we saw many Americans with Chinese babies. They stayed at the White Swan because it was next door to the only American consulate in China. The consulate issues visas, a document needed for the children to enter the United States. We felt part of a larger movement with all these Americans and their daughters.

At the White Swan we met Marco and Jackie, a couple from New Jersey who were using the same adoption agency as we were. We would be getting our daughters from the same orphanage. Peter first took us to the Office of Child Welfare, where we had to state why we wanted to adopt a baby from China and we had to promise never to hurt or abandon our child. We offered the workers gifts. We paid them $500 and received the necessary paperwork to proceed to Yangchun City, where our soon-to-be daughters were.

The next morning the four of us checked out of the White Swan to meet Peter at the train station. We searched for him in the crowded station, and when we finally met up with him, he told us about a change in plans. Instead of riding on a train with soft seats, as most foreign tourists do, we were going to ride on hard seats as most of the common people do. Three in a row were packed in as tightly as possible, with lots of bags. It was very crowded and, initially, standing room only. We would be on the train for five hours. This was the people's China, including perceptible smells. During a stop, we purchased some rice wrapped in banana leaves through the window; we took pictures of the countryside. We saw people in bare feet working in rice paddies with water buffalos, and we saw places probably quite similar to those where our daughters had been born.

Five hours later, two women from the orphanage met us at the train station. They dragged our bags to a van and drove us to the Golden Roc Hotel. It was the only hotel in this small town, and it was under renovation. The hotel had neither a coffee shop nor a restaurant. It did have a woman in the hall ready to give us hot water in thermoses for drinking. We saw no other patrons. We were taken to rather barren rooms that were next to each other. The rooms contained cribs. Peter asked us if we wanted the babies that evening, or if we wanted to wait until the next morning. We agreed to get them that evening.

After we arrived, we went out to dinner with the staff from the orphanage and Peter, who interpreted everything. We had a wonderful meal that, unexpectedly, was paid for by the director of the orphanage. After dinner, we went back to the hotel, where our babies had just arrived. It was about 8:30 p.m. The babies were strapped to the backs of their nannies. After they were passed to us, we went upstairs to our rooms, escorted by the two nannies; Mrs. Yu, the director of the orphanage; Mrs. Gao from the welfare board; and a male official. The orphanage staff stayed with us for about an hour, played with the babies, and gave us some instructions and information.

BECOMING GIANNA

Yang Jie was a very round, chubby ten-month-old from the Yang-chun City Orphanage, Guangdong Province. She and the other baby, Yang Liang (all the babies from the orphanage were given Yang as their last name), looked well cared for, and the orphanage staff was very attentive to the babies as well as to us. Since I wanted to somehow incorporate Jie's Chinese name into her American name, we named her Gianna. (Gia sounds the same as Jie.) Our new friends' child, Liang, became Arielle.

We were instructed to feed the babies a bottle four times per day: at 6 a.m., noon, 4 p.m., and 8 p.m. The bottles consisted of half dried milk and half dried rice. We mixed these dry goods with hot water. We were given a box of each to begin and were advised to keep the same food and eating schedule until we returned to the United States.

Arielle, five days older than Gia, had hair, and Gia had none. I could tell Gia was the same child from the photograph because of the shape of her ears. I had expected a tiny baby like Melody Joy, but Gia was a bit more than eighteen pounds. The size nine-month baby clothes I had brought for her were too small. We cut the feet off of the baby clothes and later bought clothes that were made in China for Chinese babies.

The manner in which the staff played with the babies was very different from how Americans play with babies. They were loud and rough and they made clicking sounds. The children responded to them positively and smiled easily. When we asked them how the selection process was made, Mrs. Yu pinched Gia's plump leg and pinched my plump leg, rubbed Gia's bald head and rubbed Joel's balding head! We have yet to hear the truth about the selection process, but there is something magical, as some parents call it, about this process. The matches are almost always perfect.

The Chinese ladies left and said they would be back the next day. We all said goodnight and closed the bedroom doors. This was our family's first night together. Joel sporadically checked on Gia, as he was afraid that she would stop breathing. After a while, we all went to sleep. The next morning, after we fed and dressed Gia and readied ourselves, we went to see how Marco, Jackie, and Arielle had done during the night. Their first night had been more intense than ours. Arielle had cried every time they had tried to lay her down.

We needed to eat breakfast, and Peter was nowhere to be found. After a short wait, we took it upon ourselves to seek out breakfast. We put the babies in Snuglis and walked out into the street. Near the hotel we noticed a sidewalk restaurant that was serving breakfast to the local people. Since there were no other options, I went to the person who seemed to be in charge and, through sign motions, told them what we wanted by pointing and holding up fingers. We ate on the plastic tables outside. We wiped our hands and mouths with the toilet paper that was provided. We ate something that looked like a cross between crepes and noodles with something inside. We drank tea. It was a fine breakfast. After we finished, we walked around a little and noticed all the people looking at us. They stopped to look at the four Caucasians with two little Chinese babies in their Snuglis. They smiled and seemed to understand what was going on. We explored Yangchun and found an open-air food market that sold live frogs and snakes, lots of vegetables, and fresh meat. Again, everyone stopped to look at us, and we just smiled.

Costs

That afternoon, the women from the orphanage returned to the hotel with a government official. It was Sunday. We needed to fill out the forms for the adoption and to give the government official $3,000. We had had to carry at least $4,000 in new 100-dollar bills to China. They had requested this because the Chinese money system is not as efficient as ours. Ten to fifteen Chinese bills equaled $100. Joel was very uncomfortable carrying that much cash, and he was relieved to hand it over to the official. We did not understand then that in China robbery of an American was severely punished.

The women continued to play with the babies. The babies were healthy and alert. It seemed as if they had been cared for adequately, which laid to rest a big fear of mine. We all went out to dinner that night (same restaurant), and this time we paid the bill.

The next day we went to the big market with Peter, before the women returned with the documents and passports. We rode in a Chinese pedicab, which was pulled by a person on foot. As soon as we arrived at the market, throngs of people gathered around us. When we stopped to eat, crowds gathered again. When they took the babies in their arms and played with them, Peter reassured us that this was all right. Personal boundaries and child safety concerns are not a part of their culture. Peter told us they were all saying what lucky babies our daughters were.

When we later met the women from the orphanage, they brought all the necessary paperwork and presents. We received a map of Yangchun City, and they marked the place on the map where our daughters had been found. Gia had been found on the side of a big street in a rice box by a man on a motorcycle who had brought her to the orphanage. Arielle had been found on the doorstep of the orphanage. They also gave us nylon stockings made in a local factory, a box of candy, which we were told was good for health, and Polaroid snapshots of the girls in the orphanage. We hugged, offered thank-yous, and said our good-byes.

Finally, we were free to leave Yangchun City. Peter explained to us that since it had rained very hard, the trains were out of service. He arranged for his friend to pick us up by van the next day to travel back to Guangzhou. One good thing that came of this van trip was that we found where the orphanage was located. We had not been invited to visit. China stopped allowing foreigners to visit the orphanages after British television aired a documentary on Chinese orphanages called *The Dying Room*. The Yangchun City Orphanage appeared to be orderly and neat from what we could see, and there were even air-conditioners in the windows. Since that time, some of the orphanages have been opened to Americans, and, in fact, privately raised American dollars are presently upgrading some of the orphanages. New relationships between the Chinese and Americans, with their adoptive children, are developing and deepening.

BEGINNING LIFE WITH GIA

We were ready to leave Yangchun for the next adventure, which turned out to be the van ride back to Guangzhou on a road that was not yet completed. China's infrastructure was still being built, and paved highways are a result of this progress. We left with Gianna and Arielle and headed for Guangzhou, another five-hour ride.

We arrived back at the White Swan and stayed for the night. The next morning we took the babies to a Chinese clinic to see a doctor for measuring and an examination. A doctor's visit was necessary before admission to the United States. We saw many Americans with adopted Chinese babies at the clinic. We had no history of Gia's health or pre-natal care. We would never be able to find out any information about Gia's birth family because abandonment of children is illegal in China, and parents can face a stiff fine (more money than a family makes in one year) if identified.

After the perfunctory examination, we said our good-byes to Marco, Jackie, Arielle, and Peter. We continued our travels for an-other week to cruise on the Yangtze River. We flew to Chongqing and were supposed to go right to the boat. A young man picked us up at the airport and told us of a change in plans. We were to stay in a hotel that night and someone would pick us up in the morning and take us to the boat. That was the night from hell. We were all alone in a hotel where no one spoke English. We were hungry and tired. There was no crib in the room and no way to get one. I went down to the fast-food restaurant in the hotel and ordered dinner by pointing. I motioned that I would take the tray upstairs. I paid for the food and went back to our room. The worst part was that Gia was crying, and although we tried, there was nothing we could do to comfort her. We walked her, talked to her, held her, put her down. We put a mattress on the floor for her. She continued to cry and scream. We did not know what else to do. Joel and I fought. It was terrible. Finally, we all got to sleep. I, being the psychotherapist, concluded that she was working out her aban-donment issues. Later we realized that Gia's problem was that she had gas pains!

In the morning a man, Mr. Lu, came to take us to the boat. He spoke English with an Oxford accent and took us out to lunch. The restaurant (similar to others in China) did not have child seats, so Mr. Lu's driver took my daughter while we ate. I asked if this was a good idea as I watched him walk my daughter out of view. Mr. Lu assured me that the driver was a good man and would not survive if he harmed an American's child. We ate. Finally, from the window I saw Gia on the man's shoulders, laughing, and she was returned to us. I came to understand that this was a customary thing—removing the child from the parents while they ate. I considered that, for the Chinese, babies must be a relative novelty since the enactment of the one-child policy.

By late afternoon, we finally got onto the boat. At dinner Gia was again taken from me so I could eat, and a female bartender played with her. It was on this boat that Gia ate tofu, her first solid food. The boat also was not "child friendly," meaning no cribs or high chairs, and our room had only two small berths, made with smaller Asian people in mind. Somehow, we endured. The scenery was magnificent, and we were saddened that the new dam the Chinese were building for flood control would flood the area by creating a large lake. Many villages would be forever lost.

After the cruise we were taken by bus to a hotel in Wuhan, where we slept well, since there was a crib waiting for Gia. As a favor to a family back in New Jersey, we carried a cash gift to be delivered to the director of the local orphanage in Wuhan, and we met him at the hotel. We then flew back to Guangzhou.

We spent our remaining days at the White Swan, and we continued to build a friendship with an English-speaking Chinese woman named Mary, whom we had met on the boat. Mary was thirty-two years old and was traveling on the Yangtze with a man younger than herself. She spoke of wanting a life of freedom and not wanting to be married, and of the difficulties of being a Chinese woman and not conforming to societal expectations. I told her about my life and how I had not conformed either. She invited us to her parents' home for dinner. We spent most of our free time with Mary, eating, sight-seeing, and shopping. She reported to us that some people on the street had asked if Gia belonged to her and Joel, who was carrying Gia in the Snugli. They assumed that Joel was her husband, because Chinese men are not seen in that kind of caretaking role.

We went to our appointment at the consulate and applied for Gia's visa. As we walked to the U.S. consulate and saw the American flag, I got very emotional as I told my daughter that we would be taking her to a country where freedom was cherished. We had to return the next day to pick up the visa, and then we would be able to leave China.

Coming Home and Being a Family

We were greeted at the airport by my family and brought home. Over the next few weeks, Gia was introduced to our family and friends through three baby showers. We were aware that her fine and gross motor skills were developmentally delayed because she could not hold anything with her fingers, and she was not crawling or pulling herself up in her crib. I applied to the New Jersey Early Intervention Program, where it was determined that she qualified for services. The waiting list for an appointment was three months, so we were given reading material on how to help her in the meantime. Joel

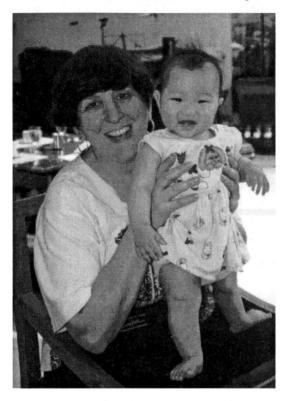

Margaret and Gianna at about eleven months old

taught her how to crawl and how to stand up in her crib. Gia seemed to respond very well to the attention and stimulation she got once she was put in our arms. By the time of the appointment for treatment, Gia at fifteen months was walking and talking, and it was obvious that she did not need services. We came to find out that many Chinese babies from orphanages have some developmental delays but catch up quickly.

Joel and I decided we would remain a three-person family, although we have been tempted to adopt a second Chinese child at times. My age seems to be an impediment. Prior to being a mother, I felt ageless because I had no benchmarks by which to measure time. This is no longer the case: when Gia turns thirteen, I will turn sixty, and when she turns eighteen, I will turn sixty-five. We are very happy being a one-child family, although Joel and I are frequently concerned about raising an only child since we both come from families with three or more siblings. We socialize with three other only-child families who have adopted from China. The girls are Gia's "Chinese sisters," and they have overnights and go on special outings together. This has become our support group and part of our chosen family.

Gia has been an easy child to raise. Her lack of stimulation in the beginning of her life has resulted in a curiosity and an interest in many things. She is very feminine, more than I ever was, and we credit that to genetics. She has known about being "made in China" since the time she began learning English. From the beginning we have incorporated her adoption story with her three friends who were also born in China. Thus, the questions she has asked are about birthing and growing babies in mommies' bellies. For example, when she was about three, she said babies are either born in hospitals (as in America) or in China (as she was). Her non-Chinese friends seem to have more questions about Gia, her adoption, and China than Gia has. So far, it appears that Gia has come to integrate her birth and her adoptive parents well.

KEEPING IN TOUCH
WITH THE CHINESE CULTURE

After five years, I finally realized that my daughter is as American as I am. The major difference is that she has a Chinese face. This fact so far has not presented any problems, but we are expecting some rough spots in the future. Because China is part of her history and race, we will continue to bring some Chinese culture into our family life. How much Chinese culture is a question many families with children from China ask themselves. Joel and I will carry the Chinese culture for her in the best way that we can until and unless she tells us to stop.

We continue to be members of Families with Children from China because we believe it is important for Gia, Joel, and me to be exposed to others living in similar situations. We attend the annual Chinese Culture Day with more than 500 families from the New York area and other special events that the group sponsors.

Our family currently observes two holidays related to Gia's Chinese heritage. The first is Family Day, which we annually celebrate with Marco, Jackie, and Arielle around April 12, the day we first met our daughters. We celebrate this holiday in different ways. Last year we went to New York's Chinatown after spending the afternoon in a botanical garden. We ate in a Chinese restaurant and the girls played in the playground across the street. The four of us, again, were the only Caucasians at the playground and restaurant. For the first time, I could not instantly spot my daughter among the other children. She blended in with the other children rather than being the only Chinese face in the crowd.

The second holiday is the Lunar New Year. In China this holiday is celebrated for two weeks with much preparation and the observation of many traditions. Since the new year is celebrated over two weeks, we have two parties. The guests at one are our dear friends, who, of course, include the three families with daughters from China. The second party is for honoring ancestors, and our blood family members are our guests.

I also have made presentations at Gia's schools about the Lunar New Year and about her birth and adoption. So far this has been acceptable to Gia. One Mother's Day we threw flowers into the river for our mothers: my mother, Gia's Grandma Mary, and Gia's birth mother. We are building a library of Chinese books, videos, stories, and scrapbooks for her.

We also made an additional attempt to bring Chinese culture into our home by inviting three Chinese exchange students to live with us. The first one was a sixteen-year-old male, who initially spoke little English. Gia's first response was that she did not want anybody Chinese talking to her or playing with her. His play with her was different from what she was used to. Until he spoke some English, it was difficult for all of us. He won her over by feeding her chocolate M&Ms, just like my mother would. Of course, it was their secret. By the time he left our home nine months later, we all loved him, and Gia regarded him as her Chinese brother. The other two students, both female, stayed a very short time and did not bond with any of us. Although Joel and I learned a lot from these experiences, we decided to stop bringing Chinese culture into our home in this way.

GIA'S ADOPTION STORY

Gia will never know her birth parents and family unless, of course, China changes its policy in her lifetime. She will never know why

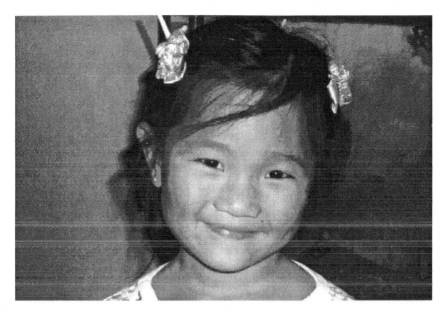

Gianna at about five years old

they could not keep her, even though it is known why most baby girls are abandoned. As preadoptive parents, we were comforted in the knowledge that we would never be legally challenged in terms of losing her. I understand, as a therapist and as her mother, that there may be a longing, a loss deep inside of her, that I will not be able to touch. How could a country of one billion people send her away? How could her birth parents make the choice to give her up? This sense of loss and rejection is something from which we cannot protect her. It is a grief I can only comfort her through if and when she feels it, and if she accepts comfort from me. Someday, Gia will be able to understand governments, societies, and policies. I have saved many articles, books, and tapes so she may understand China better, should she want to. This is the best we can do in addition to honestly and simply answering her questions as she asks them.

I used to wonder about her birth mother. As I learned more about China and its social repression, I realized that she probably never looked at her feelings about abandoning Gia. Many popular books and films, such as Amy Tan's *The Joy Luck Club,* show how difficult it is for Chinese women to look at their losses. We have told Gia that her birth mother, for reasons we will never know or understand, could not keep her and that she gave her up for adoption in the hope that someone would give her a better life than she was able to give her. My hope is that her birth mother believes that her little girl is one of the lucky ones who became part of a family that is committed to loving and caring for her always.

When I look at my daughter's Chinese face, I can see clearly that she is an individual with her own destiny. As I look into her black Chinese eyes, I am reminded that she made it from the rice box to the orphanage to the United States. I am reminded that she is, first and foremost, her own person. We are her guardians to help guide her through life to the best of our abilities. Parenting Gia has deepened our capabilities for joy and wonder, and Joel and I are amazed at the depth of our love for her. Guan Yin, the Chinese Goddess of Mercy, has truly blessed us. I want Gia to believe that she can achieve anything she chooses to and that her choices are endless. If we saved Gia from anything, it was from being a woman living in rural China like, as the old saying goes, grass to be stepped on.

REFERENCES

Kristof, N. D. and Wudunn, S. (1994). *China wakes: The struggle for the soul of a rising power.* New York: Vantage.
Tan, A. (1989). *The joy luck club.* New York: Ballantine Books.

Chapter 5

The Family I Wanted

Elizabeth Allen

I was in my thirties and living in the Washington, DC, area when the idea of adopting a child as a single parent first occurred to me. I, similar to many single women in the DC area, was working as an attorney for the federal government. My job was fully consuming, as I traveled around the United States litigating cases in the federal courts. I often worked fifty to sixty hours a week. Yet as year after year of this lifestyle continued, I felt that something was definitely missing, and I saw no likelihood that I would meet someone and marry in the increasingly short period of time I thought I had in which to start a family. At some point, I came across an article in the *Washingtonian* magazine that described the decision of a single female journalist to adopt a baby from India. I cannot tell you how important this one article was in providing the inspiration to pursue adoption. I read it many times and then filed it neatly in my filing cabinet under "Adoption."

GETTING STARTED

Finally, in the spring of 1991, I decided to pursue the adoption of a child. I was thirty-seven years old when I first contacted an organization listed in the article, the Committee for Single Parent Adoption, and several days following my call was stunned to receive in the mail a whole new world of information about adoption. I eagerly phoned and wrote to the various organizations listed in the booklet. I enrolled in a six-week adoptive parent education course run by parent volunteers. This proved invaluable in identifying potential routes to adoption and made what at first seemed to be an insurmountably complicated process doable. I rapidly progressed to contemplating the various options. Would I adopt a child domestically? Would I adopt transracially? From which countries could I, as a single woman, adopt? How much was this going to cost and how would I put together a financial plan for doing so?

At some point it became clear to me that I needed to begin the process of a home study, as this was the necessary predicate to any adoption, whether international or domestic. I contacted a social services agency recommended by several of the women I met in the single-parent adoption group and began the process of filling out numerous forms and collecting the documents required for a home study by the state of Virginia. These included my birth certificate, financial forms, and medical forms. I met with a social worker on three occasions, and she visited my home to ensure that I had carefully considered the decision to adopt and to assist me in working through the various options.

Choosing a Path—International versus Domestic Adoption

Fairly quickly, I decided that I was more comfortable pursuing an international adoption than a domestic adoption. At this point, more than ten years ago, single-parent adoptions were much less common than they are today, and I felt that I would be competitively disadvantaged, for want of a better term, as a single parent. I knew that large numbers of couples were seeking to adopt in the United States and that the climate domestically was one in which birth parents increasingly chose the adoptive parent. I could not imagine that many birth parents would choose a single-parent over a two-parent family. I considered the possibility that I, a Caucasian, would adopt an African-American child domestically but rejected that course upon learning that an African-American social workers' professional organization opposed these transracial adoptions. In addition, *The Washington Post* regularly ran articles detailing the pitfalls awaiting families who adopted children domestically only to lose them to birth parents who changed their minds or to courts who decided that it was not healthy for an African-American child to grow up with a Caucasian parent.

At the same time, my research was making me increasingly aware of countries willing to allow international adoption of children living in government-run orphanages. These countries seemed to welcome single parents. In the fall of 1991, as my home study was nearing completion, I began the process of interviewing international adoption agencies. I talked with agencies located all over the United States. I learned that almost any agency would work with me even though I lived out of state. In selecting an agency, my antennae were up for hints that an agency discriminated against single parents. If I detected anything less than enthusiasm for my inquiry, I rejected the agency. I rejected several local agencies that told me couples could express preferences for age or gender of a child but singles could not. I rejected another local agency because it was clearly uncomfortable with mothers who would continue to work outside the home following the adoption.

Selecting an International Adoption Agency

One agency that I spoke with stood out as an excellent prospect. This agency, the World Association for Children and Parents, located in Seattle, Washington, had a well-established international adoption program and expressed no reservations at all about my single status. At the time I contacted the agency in the fall of 1991, they were working with several countries that were open to single parents. Also, and more important, the week that I called the agency it had just learned that the People's Republic of China would welcome single-parent applicants in their brand-new international adoption program. They took pains to emphasize to me that the China program would be a pioneer program and, therefore, by definition untested. Nevertheless, I was impressed by what I heard and by the agency's track record and experience in setting up other successful international adoption programs. Despite the caveats, I was excited by what I heard. I simply could not believe my good fortune.

Since childhood I had been aware of adoptions of children from Vietnam and South Korea. I had read a number of books about the experiences of families who had adopted children from Asian countries in the early years of international adoption. My great-aunt had been a medical missionary in China for twenty-some years prior to the Communist revolution in the 1940s. I had grown up with Chinese objects in my home and had been very intrigued by my great-aunt's career. I also had learned in my initial forays into international adoption that Korea did not allow adoption by single parents, and at the time I was looking at options, Vietnam's program had ceased to operate for all practical purposes. When I learned that China would welcome applications by single women and that China had thousands of babies, largely girls, in state-run orphanages, I knew that I had found my program. The agency told me that it required parents to apply to more than one program at a time, as the vagaries of international adoption could derail even a well-researched and chosen adoption plan in a given country. At the time I applied to the agency, Romania's program was also willing to work with single parents, although adoptions in that country were subject to a moratorium of indeterminate length while the country altered internal procedures.

Choosing China

To adopt from the People's Republic of China, I needed to satisfy the requirements of the state of Virginia, the U.S. Immigration and Naturalization Service (INS), and the People's Republic of China. Any adoption, whether domestic or international, would require a home study. The INS would be involved because the adoption would cross international borders and the child would enter the United States as a foreign national and acquire U.S. citizenship as the adopted child of a U.S. citizen. In China, adoptions are handled solely by the Chinese government; there is no private adoption in China. The children who are available for adoption are either the documented orphans of parents who have died or, much more typically, children abandoned by their birth parents due to either the country's strict population-control policies limiting children to prescribed quotas per family, or birth defects requiring sophisticated medical treatment unavailable to the majority of the population, or, increasingly in the past ten years, having been born to unwed mothers. Whatever the reason for their status as orphans, the children have been placed in government-run children's welfare institutes to be raised. Sometimes the institutes have established foster care programs among community families, but this practice varies across the provinces. From the late 1980s, when the first international adoptions in China began, usually as a result of missionary contacts, up to 1992, when China enacted its first adoption law, to the present, international adoptions have grown from a mere handful to literally 10,000 a year. Still, the number of adoptions does not begin to address the population of children living in children's welfare institutes across the vast country.

A family living in the United States and pursuing the adoption of a Chinese child will typically spend $12,000 to $15,000 in fees for the expenses of the U.S.-based child placement agencies, the various INS fees, the required $3,000 orphanage donation, the approximately $1,000 in document-processing fees in China, and the required international flight and travel expenses associated with an approximately two-week stay in China. These fees have become very predictable and have stabilized over the past ten years. A Chinese adoption today costs no more, and in many cases less, than it did ten years ago. Families rarely encounter hidden charges as one often hears happens in other international adoptions. The process is heavily regulated by the Chinese government and, as such, is one of the most predictable international adoption programs available today.

AT LONG LAST—A DAUGHTER

I applied to adopt my first child in October 1991. I collected the documents China required, and they were sent to China in February 1992. On June 13, I received a call from the agency representative in Seattle. She told me that the China program director had received a referral of a healthy ten-week-old baby girl during her visit the previous day to the Hangzhou Children's Welfare Institute in Zhejiang Province just southeast of Shanghai. I was told that the agency director had taken photos of the baby, which I would eventually receive, but that I would first receive some very basic medical information on the baby, which had been translated from the Chinese. Shortly thereafter, I was looking at a piece of paper startling for the amount of white space—just a few measurements, a few blood test results, and the statement "healthy." The child had received an assigned name upon her entry to the orphanage, and the child's birth parents were unknown. While thrilled finally to be at the point in the process where a baby was becoming a reality, I was stunned by how little I knew and how much I had to proceed on blind faith that what I was doing was right for me. I told the agency representative that I "accepted" the referral, and this allowed the process in China to move forward with the matching up of my file with that of the baby. Approximately two weeks later I received a beautiful photo of the baby and even a minute-long video, both of which helped raise my excitement level to a near feverish pitch as I prepared to leave for China.

I arrived in Hangzhou, the provincial capital of Zhejiang province, on July 13, 1992, and met my daughter, then three and a half months old. I learned little more about her in the brief interviews with the orphanage officials than I had learned in the previous month through the first faxed medical reports. Nevertheless, I had no doubts from the time I first met her that she was a healthy baby girl, and I had complete confidence in my decision to proceed with her adoption.

My Daugher's Early Years

With the benefit of hindsight and nearly ten years of education in adoption-related issues, I now recognize that even at three and a half months my daughter displayed some classic symptoms of attachment-related difficulties. She actively resisted cuddling, she insisted on holding her own bottle, and she suffered sleep difficulties and extreme separation anxiety in the nine-month to three-year range. She had problems with self-regulation.

In addition, she was extremely strong-willed. My first year as a parent was definitely a challenge. I was chronically sleep deprived and exhausted from trying to keep up with her as she climbed to the top of the playground tower at fifteen months old, explored electrical outlets, escaped from high chairs and strollers and car seats with Houdini-like skill, and quickly emptied cupboards of all their contents. All who encountered her assured me that she was really something special! A future Olympian, they would say.

Choosing Child Care

Fortunately, I had a partner in caring for my daughter—a nanny whom I had hired shortly after returning from China. I had explored the possibility of placing my daughter in a child care center at my office, but there were no openings. I left for China with no firm plan in place. I had placed an ad for a nanny in my neighborhood newspaper the evening before I left, and when I returned, a woman had called and expressed interest. She had been with a family who had just moved to another state, so she was looking for a new position. She was young and energetic and highly experienced at child care. She came with fabulous references. I hired her and returned to work about six weeks after returning from China. I never worried that my daughter was not in good hands. My nanny fell in love with my daughter and proceeded to teach and encourage her as if she were her own daughter. Together, they set about exploring our neighborhood during the day while I was at work.

Despite having a full-time caregiver in my own home, my work life definitely changed. I no longer had complete flexibility to jump into each opportunity or crisis that presented itself, as I had someone else to consider. Fortunately, I had become a manager of attorneys in the months leading up to my daughter's arrival, a position with more predictable hours and less travel. I was able to juggle my job and parenting because I had a job that was somewhat controllable *and* I had excellent child care.

Creating a Supportive and Diverse Circle of Friends

From our earliest days as a family, I sought the friendship of other adoptive families, both single-parent and two-parent families. These included families with domestically and internationally adopted children. The children adopted internationally come from China, the former USSR, the Ukraine, Guatemala, Vietnam, and Romania. In addition, we have maintained connections with the group of families with whom we traveled to China. We have attended six biannual reunions with other China adoptive families. Because we live in an extraordinarily international community in the DC area, my children (more have been added) have had the benefit of not feeling their "differences" as profoundly as they might have had we lived in the Midwest, where I grew up. Nevertheless, I remember well the period when my eldest talked about the fact that we had no daddy in our family and another period when she actively mourned the fact that she did not grow in my tummy. In addition to being an avid reader of the adoption literature available in the popular press, so as to stay ahead of the curve on developmental issues that children typically encounter, I have emphasized that she is not alone in not having a daddy or having been adopted and that she has many friends who have the same differences within their families. Certainly, having three younger siblings with the same circumstances helps ameliorate her feelings of difference.

My Eldest Daughter Today

In the ten years that have elapsed since adopting my eldest daughter, I have survived her challenging infant and toddler years and am now enjoying watching her mature. At ten years old, she is a very bright, extremely independent child who is mature beyond her years. She has taken the extraordinary physical energy and coordination she displayed in toddlerhood and channeled it into success in competitive gymnastics and diving. She reads voraciously, is academically and musically gifted, and has a bevy of friends. She is a child to whom everything seems to come easily.

OUR FAMILY EXPANDS

In 1994, when my eldest daughter was two, I brought home her sister from China. This adoption had a new series of challenges. First, the Chinese government had abruptly closed down its international adoption program for nine long months while it reevaluated its internal policies and procedures. During that period, I considered changing countries for my second adoption and even went so far as to apply to another country for a child. I ultimately completed the process in China when the program reopened there.

New Challenges—Exploring Special Needs

In electing to proceed with a second adoption from China, I had to deal with a rule that China employed for the majority of the first decade of the program: the special needs rule. For any family that already has children, whether by birth or adoption, a subsequent child must have "special needs." The interpretation of this rule varied over the years, but when I applied to adopt my second child, I knew that I would need to be comfortable with some level of physical birth defect. I was willing to abide by this rule; other families who were not chose other programs or waited until the enforcement of the rule was more lax. In any event, I thoroughly researched various physical birth defects and ultimately accepted the referral of an adorable five-month-old baby girl with a cleft lip. I did so after learning that this birth defect is easily repaired and that the physical defect is rarely associated with more complicated syndromes. I consulted with two plastic surgeons before going to China and ultimately selected one with whom I felt comfortable. Two weeks after arriving in the United States, my daughter had her cleft lip surgically repaired, followed by insertion of ear tubes six months later. My daughter's babyhood was otherwise quite normal.

Adjusting to the Demands of Two Young Children

My second daughter was a highly affectionate child who adored her nanny as well as her mother. She was happy and on the active end of the spectrum, but not as willful or as physically busy as my eldest child. When people would ask if it really was exponentially more difficult to have two children than one, as many parents say, I would reply that, actually, this child was a breeze compared to her older sister, though perhaps having two did not seem so difficult because I was becoming a more experienced parent.

I had made the decision in building our family that I wanted the children to be close enough in age that they could be playmates. In fact, there is a twenty-two month difference between my first and second daughters, and I view that as ideal. They are close enough to share interests, yet far enough apart developmentally as to have their own spheres at any given time. Certainly, one of my greatest joys as a parent has been seeing them interact as sisters and best friends.

My Second Daughter Today

Today my second daughter has blossomed into a successful third grader. She, similar to her older sister, is a very successful student. She loves to read and is an excellent artist and athlete. She has followed her sister's footsteps in choosing competitive gymnastics, despite my best efforts to help her find an athletic niche of her own. She is an extraordinarily warm and creative child, a lover of animals, and the most determined of all my children. She is also beautiful—her cleft lip repair in no way diminishes a lovely face. Many people comment on her beauty and are unaware that she was born with a cleft.

Her life is not without its challenges. At age seven, she was diagnosed with attention-deficit hyperactivity disorder (ADHD). She now takes stimulant medication that has resulted in marked improvement in her overall functioning. In addition, we have entered a period in which her physical special needs are requiring greater day-to-day attention, as she has begun significant orthodontia. We are working with an orthodontist who specializes in craniofacial issues; he is working to encourage her undersized upper jaw to grow to bring it into proper alignment with her lower jaw. In addition to having a palate expander appliance and braces, she wears nightly headgear to assist in correction of the structure of her jaw. I am extraordinarily proud of the matter-of-fact way she handles her challenges.

TAKING THE PLUNGE ONCE AGAIN

In 1996, our family expanded to include my third daughter. While my life with two young children, one of whom had some special needs, was certainly challenging, I felt confident that another child would add greater richness to our lives. I began the adoption process with the plan to adopt a non-special needs infant, as that option was then open to me. Nevertheless, my plan changed when I learned about a specific child with physical special needs who was living in the orphanage from which a friend's children had come.

Embracing Special Needs

My daughter was fourteen months old when I first learned of her, and she had already had one surgery in China to repair a defect of the intestinal tract. I was told that even though she was a beautiful little girl with a very engaging personality that drew people to her, the orphanage viewed the child as essentially unadoptable due to her birth defect, which might mean that she would never have normal bowel control. Never one to walk away from a challenge, I undertook to learn everything I could about this particular birth defect and the prospects for repairing or treating it here in the United States. Through the wonders of the Internet, I learned of a support group of parents with children born with similar conditions, and my contacts with that group led me to a world-renowned surgeon practicing in suburban New York City who had invented the surgical technique then viewed as state of the art for correcting the birth defect. I contacted the surgeon and provided him with as much medical information as I had been able to gather about the child. I asked for a prognosis and was told that she would need additional surgery here in the United States and that it was possible that, with time, she would have normal bowel function. I was clearly told, however, that it was also possible that she would not achieve normal bowel function, and the worst-case scenario was that she would need a daily enema for the rest of her life. While I had gone into the process of exploring the adoption of a special needs child with the thought that I could say no if I found that her needs were more than I could comfortably take on, I discovered along the way that I wanted to adopt this child, whatever her medical prospects.

I left for China to adopt my third daughter only forty-eight hours after being informed that I had the approval of the Chinese government to travel. I had been working on various contingent travel plans for several weeks and so was poised to travel, literally, at a moment's notice. I left my two young children in the care of my trusted nanny. My mother and I traveled to meet my new daughter, then eighteen months old. This was my first adoption of a toddler and I was somewhat apprehensive about how easily she would accept me. I took my mother along to assist me if we had a particularly difficult time initially due to my daughter's older age. We learned quickly that, for whatever reason, this child would be the easiest child in my family. She was exceptionally sweet and quiet in the first days but rapidly began opening up. She loved the stacking cups we brought and played with them—clearly the first toys she had ever had—intently for hours at a time. She ate and slept well and handled the additional ten days in China with ease. Although she was only seventeen pounds at eighteen months and her leg muscles were poorly developed, it was clear that she would overcome these delays in due course. For the first time I returned from China quite well rested.

Navigating the Surgery and Treatment Maze

The first months following our return were among the most difficult of my parenting years to date. I took my daughter for several days of medical tests both in my hometown and ultimately in suburban New York City. Within a month of our return I had moved the entire family and my nanny into the Ronald McDonald house adjacent to the hospital for what would be a two-and-a-half-week stay. My surgeon had determined that my daughter had likely been born with a relatively minor form of the intestinal defect but that a surgical repair would be required to give her the best chance of achieving full bowel control. A surgical slot had become available and they could do the surgery within a week. My daughter weathered the surgery and the two weeks of being fed intravenously with her customary equanimity. I, on the other hand, found being in a hospital for eighteen days, twenty-four hours a day, a recipe for rapid insanity. I was exhausted from lack of sleep and from participating in the medical stresses of my daughter's many roommates. I will say that ministering to a sick child is a great way to enhance the bonding process.

We returned to suburban Virginia during the dog days of August, and life achieved some normalcy in September when my older two daughters returned to preschool and I returned to my job. For the next two years, I held my breath as I dealt with postsurgical therapies and medication, alternating bouts of constipation and diarrhea, and ultimately potty training. I am delighted to say that by age four my daughter had near normal bowel control and was fully self-sufficient.

My Third Daughter Today

My daughter is now a happy second grader. She has an amazingly sweet and sunny personality. She is a true friend to each of her classmates and shows powers of observation and analysis much beyond her years. She is also extraordinarily independent, perhaps a vestige of her first eighteen months of life when she had to manage everything on her own. She has just completed a highly successful week of sleep-away camp at the tender age of seven, an experience she begged for at length before I gave in.

Her life is not without challenges. She takes a daily laxative to counter the effects of her birth defect and subsequent surgery. She will likely do so for the rest of her life. In addition, she is entering her third year of speech therapy to address some oral motor weakness and articulation issues. These are likely a vestige of her first eighteen months in the orphanage when she drank from bottles that had large slits cut in them to facilitate fast feeding. This led to underdeveloped muscles in her mouth that have affected her speech, albeit no more than many children of more typical beginnings.

She is a delightful child who experiences life with such gusto that it would be easy to forget that she came to me with significant special needs. When I think that she was once viewed as "unadoptable," I am reminded that no child should ever be viewed in this way, and I know that I would feel this way whether or not her birth defect had been able to be remedied.

AND THEN THERE WERE FOUR

For the next four years following the addition of my third daughter, our lives were very busy. I became accustomed to hearing that old adage "You certainly have your hands full" at least once a day. In the first years following my older daughters' adoptions I had seemed constantly to be dealing with unwanted attention from others in public and with the fairly constant inquiry, "Are they really sisters?" With three young children and one parent, I had learned to ignore most of the intrusive questions, as there was always a child who needed to be chased and I simply had no time to get stuck in a conversation about our family origins. It was a period of coming to terms with now being viewed as a larger family. At some point I realized that I no longer even cared about what people thought of my highly unusual family. I now recognize this as the point at which it became possible to think of adopting again.

Deciding to Add a Fourth Child

The year my youngest daughter entered full-day kindergarten I noticed a definite if subtle difference in the parental demands. My children were finally at the age where it seemed I could read the newspaper and drink a cup of coffee on a weekend morning while they played in the basement, without constant fear that they were endangering their lives when out of my sight. So when I announced, only six weeks before traveling, to my family and closest friends that I was adopting again, there was a quite audible gasp: "But it is just getting manageable. Are you crazy?"

Applying to Adopt a Specific Child

As rich as my life had been for the nine years since the arrival of my eldest daughter, I had for several years been struggling with the sense that our family was not yet complete. Finally, in the summer of 2000, a good friend traveled to China and visited my third daughter's orphanage. Knowing that I had recently launched a plan to adopt a fourth child, she called me from China to say that she had found him. He was two years old and a beautiful, healthy little boy who had recently come into the orphanage!

Contrary to popular belief, about five percent of the children in the children's welfare institutes in China are boys. They are available for adoption for the full range of reasons that children are available for adoption everywhere. Some are true orphans whose parents have died; many have physical handicaps; and some are the children of young, unwed mothers.

I contacted the agency that had placed my third daughter with me and asked them to represent me in requesting that this little boy be assigned to my family. Thus began the fourth scramble to pull together a "dossier" to send to China that would be my application for the adoption of this child. In August 2000, I mailed my dossier to China and then began a six-month wait to see if the authorities would agree that I could adopt this little boy. It was not easy to wait for word when I already had photos of the child and could easily visualize this little boy spending the cold winter in an orphanage, albeit an orphanage I already knew and respected. In February 2001, as the entire family was at home with the stomach flu, I learned that the Chinese Center for Adoption Affairs had agreed that I could adopt him. I traveled in late March 2001 to China, accompanied by my eldest daughter, to bring him home.

Bringing Home an Older Child

I elected to bring my eldest daughter with me to China to adopt my son because I thought it would be helpful to him in making the transition to our family. After all, her Chinese face would be a comfort to him and her acceptance of me would demonstrate to him that he need not be afraid, and, in fact, that is pretty much how it went. My son readily accepted his new sister. She sat patiently in the orphanage conference room offering him toys and food and holding him on her lap, and when the moment came for me to hold him, his stoicism collapsed and he cried uncontrollably. He soon recovered, however, and accepted me somewhat warily while continuing to accept his sister's attentions with greater enthusiasm.

Our stay in China was not particularly difficult. My son cried little and had relatively few tantrums. He loved the food, the toys, the bath, and his sister. Of course, once we arrived home, real life intervened and things became decidedly more challenging. He developed a lot of control issues, not surprising for a child who had lost all control at the tender age of two years. He was amazingly stubborn and willful and would shriek and carry on uncontrollably when things did not go his way. His sisters announced often and loudly that they would have preferred a baby—preferably a girl—instead of this loud, obnoxious, demanding boy. Through a year of difficult adjustments, we survived and somehow things have gradually improved.

My Son Today

He has now been home for seventeen months. He is an amazing little boy. He has thoroughly bonded with our family. His first question upon waking in the morning is "Where's guys?"—referring to his three sisters. He demands kisses—three kisses—from Mom as I leave for work, and he asks each day, "You pick me up from school, OK?" He went to preschool every morning this past year and managed it well. He has fabulous gross motor skills and loves any playground or swimming pool. He loves books and all kinds of toy vehicles. His language skills are exploding and I hear new words and sentences each day. He can write his name, swim under water, jump off a diving board, and brush his teeth (finally). He has thoroughly turned our lives on end, but we are adjusting to him and he to us. He has just turned four years old.

SUGGESTIONS FOR THOSE CONTEMPLATING A LARGER FAMILY

What can I offer to those who are thinking about adopting multiple children?

1. *Take it one step at a time.* I did not go into the adoption of my first daughter thinking that I would adopt four children. It happened over a ten-year period and with significant periods for adjustment be-

tween each adoption. My second adoption followed the first by exactly two years and the third followed the second by another two years. My last adoption followed the third by almost four years. I have friends who adopted several children simultaneously, but I think that is extremely challenging for a single parent. It was very helpful to me to be able to concentrate on the adjustment of one new child at a time. Of course, each child in the family makes adjustments to the newly configured family as well.

2. *Identify your strengths as a parent in contemplating additions to your family.* At each point in the process of considering adding a child, I asked myself what I had to offer a child. In my case, as a single working parent, I was not able to offer a mom who was at home during the day. I therefore decided that I was not a good fit for a child with major special needs who needed lots of one-on-one attention. Nor was I, in my mind, a good fit for a much older child who would have significant educational and language deficits that would require much time and attention to address, as I would not be there during the homework hour. On the other hand, in the early years I counted as my assets my wonderful nanny who was especially good with babies, excellent medical insurance, and access to premier medical care in a large city. These latter assets were significant considerations in my willingness to take on minor to moderate correctable medical needs. Some people have large and supportive families living nearby; others have work schedules that allow for greater flexibility in spending time with children during the day. Each family's resources are unique.

3. *Reach out to other families and parents for support.* Single parenthood does not need to be lonely. Shortly after I adopted my first daughter, six other single adoptive parents and I established a friendship that is now ten years strong. We meet every other month or so for an adult dinner and at other times with our children. Through the years these friendships have been invaluable to me, as we have together confronted the joys and difficulties of single parenthood. In addition, I have made good friends with other families on my children's sports teams, at my children's school, in my neighborhood, and at my church. In addition, we have a number of friends from our China travel groups and we continue to see these people periodically, although we live all over the United States and world. These relationships are important to me and to my children. I believe that children benefit from concentric circles of friendship and affiliation—their

families, their teams, their schools, their churches, and their reunion groups.

4. *Accept that, as the single parent of a larger family, time will be a precious resource.* You will not be able to do everything you once did. You will not be able to keep up with every friendship from a time when your hands are less full. Your house will not look like *House Beautiful,* you will always have a very long "to-do" list, and many things will get done "just in time" and not a minute before. This is the reality. Acceptance of this reality will make your very full days more rewarding.

5. *Know that you will need to spend a lot of time tending the economics of a larger family.* I shop the half-price sales at the grocery stores, use lots of coupons, and hold every store's bonus card. My children wear hand-me-downs. Our entryway has a new box of clothes from a friend or relative nearly every month. I welcome and embrace this—it is absolutely necessary—and I am thankful for all contributions. I am extremely cost conscious, and that is OK. I view the work I do to feed and clothe my family on a budget as the price I pay for the blessing of having the family I always wanted.

Chapter 6

Our Daughters from China Have Two Mommies

Tina Morris
Lee Jones

Our family consists of two moms and two adopted Chinese daughters. We are, obviously, a nontraditional family. We live in a large city in the southeastern United States. Tina attended Harvard University and moved to New York City to attend Columbia Medical School. Lee attended Yale University and moved to New York to attend New York University School of Law. We met in New York while attending medical school and law school, respectively, and stayed in the New York City area through the completion of school, and through Tina's internship and residency while Lee worked as an attorney.

We had always dreamed of having a family and knew from the first night we met that we both desperately wanted children. We decided to leave New York City to give our children the kind of nonurban childhood we each had enjoyed. We moved south so that Tina could finish a child psychiatry residency while Lee worked as an attorney at a large national law firm.

When we were both thirty-two years old, we began the process of trying to get pregnant through alternative insemination using an unknown donor. The process was not successful. We endured several years of infertility treatments, including hormonal treatments, daily shots, and ultrasounds, and decided to stop short of in vitro fertilization. We had spent thousands of dollars with no reward, but our desire to have children had not lessened.

The authors have used pseudonyms and have chosen not to identify the agencies involved in their adoptions to protect their family's privacy.

MAKING THE DECISION TO ADOPT

We examined our feelings about having a child with biological connections to one of us versus adopting a child. We quickly concluded that having a child in our lives was far more important than any biological connection. We truly felt that our lives would not be complete without a child and that we had a lot to offer a child.

Given the nontraditional nature of our relationship, we believed that domestic adoption was not a realistic option. We had heard traumatic stories, in the media and in court cases, of biological parents regaining custody of a child after years of placement in an adoptive home that was later discovered to be "homosexual." We felt more comfortable with a closed adoption to avoid our vulnerability to that potential problem.

Recognizing that our child or children would live in an all-female household, we decided that it would be easier for us to raise girls. We wanted to adopt as young a child as possible so that we could watch her grow up and master each developmental milestone. As a child psychiatrist, Tina felt strongly that we could have a bigger impact and ensure a more secure attachment if we adopted an infant.

Shortly before we made our decision to adopt, a good friend of ours who is Chinese American attended the International Women's Conference in Beijing. She later visited us and told us about all the female babies abandoned in China because of China's rule allowing couples to have only one child. She told us how wonderful the girls in the orphanages were and how much they needed good homes. Another friend of ours was living in Mongolia and working in an orphanage there. She and her husband had adopted four Mongolian children.

At the time we were considering adopting from China, we met several couples, including some female couples, who had returned from China with healthy infants. After one look at the beautiful, smiling faces of those babies, we knew that we should adopt a Chinese girl. We sought the couples' advice in choosing an adoption agency. Many very good agencies specialize in international adoptions and several specialize in the adoption of children from China. In the end, we chose a private, nonprofit agency that specialized in Chinese adoptions.

THE ADOPTION PROCESS:
A CIRCUITOUS PAPER CHASE

The entire adoption process was both exciting and emotionally draining. As with most major life changes, it required a good bit of hard work, patience, and faith. As we began the process, we encountered people, agencies, and procedures of which we had never before been aware. Because our adoption agency was located out of state, we had to choose a local agency for the completion of our adoption home study. The process of adoption was unique for us. Tina adopted as a single parent. Even so, the local agency was very thorough in evaluating the suitability of both of us to be parents. We both completed the lengthy questionnaire that asked numerous questions about our lives and our motivations for becoming adoptive parents. The questions were designed to expose differences between couples in approaches to discipline, nurturing, developmental hurdles, spirituality, and a host of issues likely to arise in parenting. The process of completing the questionnaires allowed us to examine and discuss a unified approach. It was a valuable tool in accepting each other as parents, and one that we would recommend to all couples thinking of having children.

We had three interviews (two individual interviews and one as a couple) with a very warm and clinically astute licensed clinical social worker. She tried to be very inclusive and respectful of Lee's role in the process. During the home study process, Tina began gathering all the paperwork necessary for the dossier that would be sent to China. We had to get Immigration and Naturalization Service (INS) approval, which required fingerprinting and FBI background checks for both of us. We both had to have complete physical examinations and extensive blood work, including HIV testing, syphilis and hepatitis screening, and general lab work. We had to provide extensive financial statements and proof of employment. Tina also had to get several letters of recommendation.

Many of the documents had to be notarized, certified, and authenticated by the secretary of state and then the Chinese Consulate. We both came to refer to this part of the adoption process as the "paper chase." Once we had each document in hand, we would mail it to various places for its next processing and sit back and hope it would get back to us in time for the next deadline. We joked that Federal Express should have sent us a dividend check at the end of the year because we had used their services so often to expedite and ensure delivery. In many ways the paperwork process became a metaphor for pregnancy. Anything that went wrong would slow up the process and endanger the delivery of our baby to us. Needless to say, as a doctor and a lawyer, we were a bit compulsive about the paper trail.

When we started the paper chase to adopt Lia, we knew that the Chinese Adoption Center (CAC) required applicants to be at least thirty-five years old to adopt a healthy infant. At that time, Tina was only thirty-four but would turn thirty-five in January. In light of the age requirement, we completed our paperwork over roughly six months' time. We anticipated that we could send our dossier to China just after Tina's birthday. Everyone estimated that we could be through the process and have our baby girl in nine to twelve months total.

What we had not anticipated was a change in the political organization of the Chinese adoption process. This occurred in October 1996, or about halfway through our application process. The CAC made changes to the age and existing child requirements for adoptive families qualifying to receive healthy or older children as opposed to special needs children. As the CAC developed the list of special medical conditions qualifying as "special needs," all adoption processing was suspended. The international agency that handled our adoption dossier, child match, travel, and adoption finalization was extraordinary. The agency considered no question too trivial and kept us up to date and informed during the entire process.

Our dossier was sent to China by our agency in February 1997, and then the wait for our child match began. We had requested a healthy infant, but the exact age and location would be decided by the date our dossier was received.

In mid-November 1997, Tina received a phone call informing her that a baby girl had been matched with her application. The next day we received a photo and medical history. We still get very emotional recalling our excitement and anticipation on that day. Of course, we immediately fell in love with the beautiful little girl we would call Lia, who was by then ten months old. The photo we received was taken when Lia was about two and a half months old and corresponded to the date of the physical exam report. The medical information was very brief and reported that everything was "normal," including HIV testing and hepatitis screening.

The match form stated that Lia was residing in an orphanage called Maoming Children's Welfare House in Maoming City, Guangdong Province, in the People's Republic of China. She had been in the orphanage, not in foster care, for her entire infancy. As is the case with almost all baby girls adopted from China, we learned later that Lia was abandoned in the public marketplace, where she was easily discovered and taken to the Welfare Court of Maoming City for delivery to the orphanage.

The international adoption agency asked for Tina's approval of the match. She signed the form and sent it back overnight, indicating the new name that we would give to our daughter. There was never any question about our instantaneous attachment and bonding to that one little picture. Lee enlarged the picture and made a huge quantity of copies, and we gave or mailed them to all our family and friends in our Christmas cards. Everyone was so excited for us. We still have the framed 5-by-7 photo in our home, and Lia refers to it fondly as the "baby Lia picture."

Later, when we were traveling in China and everyone was regaling the group with their "match receipt" stories, we asked the in-China representative from our agency whether families ever turned down a child match. We learned that this does happen very infrequently, sometimes because of medical concerns, and that those children who are rejected are never reconsidered for adoption again. They remain in the orphanage until they are old enough to leave as adults.

We were very excited to learn that Lia was from Maoming. We had friends who had just returned six months earlier from Maoming with their adopted daughter, and they had very good things to say about the health and development of babies from the Maoming Orphanage. They asked us to bring photos of their daughter to share with the orphanage director and staff in China. In the Chinese adoption community, such ties are often described as "red threads" that tie each of us to our daughters, to her birthplace and culture, and to one another as a group of new international families. These red threads were already working to tie us firmly to our new daughter in China.

Soon we would be in China meeting our new daughter and becoming instant parents. The days passed quickly but were very busy. We were told that we would travel during the first two weeks of January 1998. A couple of weeks before we were to travel, the agency gave us some updated information about Lia. It seemed she had not grown much since her first picture and medical exam. She was reported to be only fourteen pounds. We were alarmed at how far off from the growth chart average she seemed to be. We discovered that there is a different growth chart for Asian children born and residing in Asia. We plotted her statistics on that growth chart and learned that she was still only in the tenth percentile. Rather than fret over her size, we took everyone's encouragement to heart and determined to get Lia home as quickly as possible so that we could "fatten her up." We received tremendous encouragement and support from our families, friends, and church.

The entire adoption process that we began in August 1996 spanned one and a half years. It cost roughly $12,000 in total, and we consider it the best investment we have ever made. The expenses were itemized for us in some of the very first literature we received from both our in-state and out-of-state agencies. The travel expenses and money needed for fees were spelled out in detail in our travel notice. The majority of the expenses were fees to the International Adoption Agency, totaling $3,300, a mandatory $3,000 child-rearing fee paid to the local Chinese orphanage, and a $1,200 child-placement fee paid to the Chinese central and local governments. The travel expenses for two people included round-trip airfare to China, all travel in China, and all accommodations and totaled about $3,500 for a fourteen-day trip. In addition, we paid approximately $1,000 to our local adoption agency for our home study.

People talk about love at first sight, and we understood completely when we first laid eyes on Lia. Our group received our babies in the lobby of the government office. The nannies brought the children in, and all of us excited, soon-to-be parents tried to match faces with the photos we had received so many months before. By the time they got to us, we had already spotted Lia. She was being held by the orphanage director and was quiet and content.

They called out Lia's Chinese orphanage name, and Tina went up and took her in her arms. We both were ecstatic. Lia did not cry at all but searched our faces in a very inquisitive manner, checking us out as we held her. From the government office, we were all to go to lunch and learn about the orphanage and our daughters' schedules. This was vital information for all of us novice parents. We learned that the girls had been awakened from their morning naps, dressed hurriedly, and rushed onto the bus to get to us. We then noticed that in her haste to deliver Lia to us, the nanny had put Lia's clothes on her backward. The retelling of that fact has delighted Lia ever since. Lia was extremely quiet and lethargic, and she stared fixedly without making good eye contact through lunch, prompting Tina to worry that she was autistic. By the time we made it to the bus, Lia was fully awake, smiling, and laughing at being lifted in the air. We had already had our first lesson in being worried parents and in realizing that sometimes too much medical/psychiatric knowledge can be a bad thing.

The next few days in China were a whirlwind of learning how to be parents, especially in a country where the water was not potable, the food was unknown to us, the air was not clean, the members of our travel group were all succumbing to sickness, and all three of us were staying in one small hotel room without a crib. Lia was eleven days shy of her first birthday but was drinking only formula, straight or mixed with some of the sweetest rice cereal powder we had ever tasted. She drank these "meals" from a bottle. She was thrown off her schedule in our travels and became dehydrated. She ended up constipated and required a trip to the hotel doctor for an herbal suppository.

LIA: OUR FIRST DAUGHTER

Lia was extremely petite, weighing just under sixteen pounds. Like many of the children, Lia had several scabs on her face and scalp, several bites or rash marks on her body, and a mild case of diaper rash. We treated her for scabies prophylactically and the diaper rash cleared up. Right from the start Lia had a great temperament and a wonderful smile. She slept pretty well but was difficult to feed. She would not take any solid food for some time after we returned to the United States. Lia's favorite toy was an Elmo "CD player" that played various types of music when she pushed a button. She rocked her body in time with the music. She quickly learned how to make the music work so that she could "dance." We affectionately called her musical rocking the "Maoming shuffle." When we got home, Lia delighted her grandparents with her performance. Lia also enjoyed her reflection in the mirror.

In the week we spent with Lia in China, she progressed from just barely sitting up to crawling and pulling herself up while holding onto the side of the bed. With her newfound progression to being up-right, Lia discovered that she could do the Maoming shuffle to music while standing. Some of the other children in the group began walking during the first week. We realized that all the stimulation the girls were getting was helping them catch up on motor skills rapidly. Lia walked at thirteen months, just one month after we returned home.

Lia was not talking or saying any Chinese words when we first got her. We began to talk to her in English, calling her by her new name, Lia, and she seemed to recognize it quickly. She loved to be picked up and raised high in the air. During our week in China, we taught Lia to ask us to be lifted by raising her hands in the air as we said "up." This was our first real mode of communication, and Lia loved it. It made us feel very proud of her and of ourselves. The accomplishments that induced in us such great pride in our daughter and in ourselves may seem minor, but for us they were major steps in becoming parents. Lia had bonded and attached to us without difficulty. The ten days we spent with Lia in China, concentrating solely on caring for her, made us an "instant family."

Lia resembled a typical one-year-old getting a thrill out of manipulating her environment and finding a way for her parents to meet her needs and desires. Of course, as a child psychiatrist, Tina had to be careful not to overinterpret any particular behavior or expression as a problem. Tina's initial concern about developmental delay was slowly erased, although new diagnoses sprang to mind often as we concluded our second week of travel in China. Lia caught a cold. Lee developed a severe upper respiratory infection that settled into her voice box for several weeks. Tina got a bad case of ringworm after having a pair of pants washed in the hotel laundry. As the last American Consulate interview was completed in Guangzhou and the group prepared for departure to home, we were ready to return to our comfortable Western life.

The initial few weeks home from China were busy and tiring. We had to adjust to a thirteen-hour time change and recuperate from jet lag after flying for twenty-four hours. We had to switch all of our schedules slowly from day to night. To help in this monumental time adjustment, Lee's parents eagerly met us at the airport and stayed for two weeks. Their help made adjustment to our new family life a joy.

We arrived home at about 5:00 a.m. and took Lia to her first pediatric appointment later that day. The pediatrician determined that Lia was so small that she did not make the charts for height, weight, or head size. Lia's records indicated that she had received all her shots, but blood work called that assumption into question. As a precaution, Lia was reimmunized in the United States. We slowly began to switch Lia over to American formula, then to milk and rice cereal, and finally to baby food.

She took weeks to open her mouth enough to take a spoonful of baby food. We tried giving her Cheerios, but she refused to put them in her mouth. Instead, she discovered that Cheerios make great tiddlywinks and delighted in shooting them around the house. To this day mealtime and eating are not something Lia is particularly enthusiastic about. At age five, she is still very petite but tremendously strong. She has almost no fat on her body, weighing only thirty-two pounds, and is just shy of three and a half feet tall. We were thrilled that she finally made the American growth chart for height and weight at her five-year checkup.

Lee stayed home full-time after Lia's adoption. We felt strongly that having a parent at home full-time would help any transitions Lia needed to make, and we were lucky to be able to afford to sacrifice one of our salaries. Lee returned to work part-time right after Lia's fifth birthday.

Lia began attending a nonprofit preschool program when she was about twenty months old. She was precocious and was placed in the two-year-old class, two mornings each week. The next year she attended the three-year-old class, three mornings a week, and went to five mornings a week at age four. This year she is in prekindergarten five days a week. Lia has had constant stimulation both at home and in school. She enjoys and excels at art, loves sports, and plays with many friends. She has a remarkable imagination.

Lia has become a very social, outgoing, empathic, and assertive little girl with a great sense of humor. Although she weighs only thirty-two pounds, she is solid muscle. She easily traverses the monkey bars, lifts more than her own body weight, and swings a mean T-ball bat. She has lots of friends, and her teachers report that classmates fight over who will sit next to her during school activities. She is very intelligent, eager to read, and consumed with learning other languages. She is warm, compassionate, and very affectionate. Lia has also become a model big sister to her adoptive sister, Amy.

THE DECISION TO ADOPT AGAIN: GETTING AMY

We had such a positive experience with Lia's adoption that six months after our return from China we began discussing a return trip to adopt another little girl. Both of us came from families with three children. We felt strongly that giving Lia a sister with whom to play, fight, and share the ups and downs of life would be important. We realized that our girls might be stigmatized or picked on because they had been interracially adopted into our nontraditional two-mom family. We hoped somehow that these emotionally charged issues would be tempered or buffered if we had two daughters to overcome their isolation among peers by sharing the same issues with each other.

Shortly before we adopted our second daughter, Amy, when Lia was only two and a half years old, we attended a party for several families. Many of the families were traditional two-parent, heterosexual, nuclear families. Lia sat to the side sulking. When we asked what the problem was, Lia replied that she was "sad and mad and had been for a very long time, because [she] had no dad." Over the next couple of weeks and often since then we have discussed all the different kinds of families that exist and all the ways that they are made. We celebrate our family's nontraditional makeup. As parents, we are grateful that Lia and her sister will be able to share these feelings with each other. We have continued to discuss the issue whenever either of the girls asks, and Lia has helped her little sister to be very accepting of our nontraditional family.

Lia was thrilled about getting a baby sister from China. She wondered aloud whether "baby Amy" would enjoy every activity we undertook. During the course of every new experience we tried, Lia would opine about what baby Amy would have done if she were with us. Lia also read all the books about being a big sister and dreamed of all the things she would teach her and do with her.

In September 1998, we began the paper chase for our second Chinese adoption with the same out-of-state and local agencies. The paperwork process went much more smoothly the second time around; after all, we had become "experts." There was less anxiety but the same anticipation. The major decision we had to make was how our family would travel to China. We anticipated that we would travel in late summer or early fall of 1999. Lia was only two and a half years old and too young to travel that far. We also did not think she would do well with avoiding drinking half her bathwater, and the water in China is not potable. Lee's mother offered to stay with Lia while we traveled to China for Amy, but we worried that Lia would feel left out and have problems adjusting to the arrival of her new baby sister if she were left alone without either of her moms. We sought advice over the Internet from the many people who had completed a second adoption with our agency.

We knew that Tina would have to travel again because she was the official adoptive single parent on the application. During a family vacation with Lee's parents, we first broached the idea of Lee's mom traveling to China in Lee's place. We explained the advice we had received from families who found that their first daughter was very angry and resentful when both parents left her to travel to China to adopt a second child. After learning the details of the shots required and recalling the rigors of the trip we had described the first time, Grandma agreed to go to China. Lee told Lia that she would stay home with her to prepare for the arrival of her baby sister. Lee and Lia planned many projects, including painting a child's rocking chair for Amy and picking out a new stuffed animal for her.

Tina received the phone call identifying our new daughter and promising that the photo and physical exam report would arrive the next day. Lee and Lia were visiting Lee's parents two hours away. Upon receiving the news that the match had been made, they drove home, received the Federal Express package with Amy's picture and exam, made the necessary copies of the pictures of all sizes, and returned to Grandma's with all the information. From that day on, the family began learning about Amy's home province and home city and anticipating Amy's arrival.

Tina, Lee, and Lia prepared a small, soft, baby-proof photo album filled with pictures of Amy's adoptive family. The pictures showed family members eagerly awaiting Amy's arrival. Our favorite photo, which also would become Amy's favorite, was a picture of Lia holding up Amy's match report with the photo of baby Amy. A few weeks later, Tina and Grandma got instructions for traveling to China in September 1999. Many of the families who were traveling to China in the planned group were also adopting their second Chinese daughter, so the anxiety level of the whole group was markedly less than Tina had encountered on the first trip. The itinerary and costs were all explained just as they had been on the first trip. The whole adoption process cost slightly more because of increased INS fees in the United States and because travel was at a premium at that time of year. Still the entire cost, for all fees, travel, costs in China, and all aspects of the adoption, was about $15,000.

Tina traveled with Grandma to China to bring Amy home. Amy was in Yue Yang City, in Hunan Province in the People's Republic of China. The county seat for the province is Changsha, so the group flew internationally to Hong Kong, took a bus ride to Guangzhou, and immediately flew to Changsha. Much of the process was the same, and Tina got reacquainted with the in-country staff of the agency whom she had met on the first trip. Tina shared pictures of Lia with the staff. They were all thrilled to see her and claimed to remember her well. The main difference in the second trip to China was that baby Amy was quite sick when we first got her. Amy had severe respiratory problems within the first twelve hours of our receiving her. Tina spent the early morning of her first day with Amy, from 2:00 a.m. until 6:00 a.m., in a Chinese hospital emergency room watching a nurse try to place a scalp IV into Amy's head to administer medications. Tina realized that Amy had recently been on IV medications which had made her arm and leg veins inaccessible. She also recognized healing scalp wounds from previous IV sites.

Tina was exhausted when she returned to the hotel from the hospital. Both Tina and Amy were traumatized by the ordeal and had not experienced an ideal first day together. Grandma had packed the bags in preparation for the three-and-a-half-hour bus ride they would all have to take that morning. Tina ate breakfast quickly but then threw up all of it because of her anxiety. Both Tina and Grandma had communicated with Lee and Lia about Amy's poor health and all the new difficulties they were experiencing in China. Lee worried and felt desperate to provide some help to her new daughter. She called their American pediatrician to provide some advice to Tina. We all realized that we just needed to get baby Amy through the trip and get her home. Lee and Lia discussed that Amy was sick, but they agreed with Tina and Grandma that they were all thrilled and thankful that Amy was finally part of their family.

In China, the group left Changsha to travel by bus to Yue Yang City, where Amy's orphanage was located. Amy was still very sick on the ride, and Tina feared she would not make it. Because of construction and a flat tire, the trip in ninety-five-degree weather on a bus without air-conditioning lasted almost six hours. On the evening that they arrived, Tina and Grandma learned that baby Amy had recently been hospitalized for asthma and treated with prednisone, a very strong steroid, and aminophylline. The nanny had forgotten to bring the medications for Amy. A nurse who had taken care of Amy in the Yue Yang orphanage was sent late that night to deliver the medicine.

The orphanage in Yue Yang was under renovation at the time, so the group did not get to visit. The nannies and orphanage director brought each child a nice box of gifts, including a videotape of the child's early months at the orphanage. We also received the outfit that Amy was wearing when she was found, and pictures of her orphanage, her nanny, and her life in the orphanage. We feel fortunate to have this early infant history for Amy. Since the time that we brought Amy home with all of this personal information and history, we have managed to get some pictures of Lia in her orphanage with her nanny. These snapshots of their lives in China have become a favorite topic of conversation and comparison in the girls' "recollections" of their birthplaces.

Amy got better within twenty-four hours of receiving her medicine in Yue Yang. By the time the group returned to Changsha the next day, Amy was showing her spirit and proving to be a handful. Upon regaining some strength, Amy immediately exhibited her voracious appetite. She shocked her mother and grandmother on several occasions by screaming at the top of her lungs until they shared large portions of their meals with her. Amy had no hesitation about eating solid food and had little interest in accepting a meal from a bottle. She proved to have a challenging independent streak that we have fought hard not to label as "stubborn" or "hardheaded." She also knew, even at nine months, how to throw a temper tantrum.

When we first brought Amy home, she was firmly attached to Tina and Grandma. She was scared of Lee and often upset, although intrigued, by Lia. She adapted to the time difference fairly quickly and felt comfortable enough with Tina and Lee that we sent Grandma home with Grandpa after only four days. To this day, Amy has a fierce attachment to her grandmother and often voices how much she misses her, even in the middle of participating fully in a fun event. Amy idolizes her big sister. She plays copycat to Lia so often that we are amazed when we lose patience with this practice long before Lia does.

After engaging in monumental struggles over Amy's temper tantrums, Lee and Amy have developed a very strong bond, and Amy has really gotten control of her anger. She now has an impish personality and a fiendishly delightful belly-rolling laugh. She loves slapstick, physical humor but comprehends and enjoys her sister's more subtle wordplay humor. Amy is incredibly bright, thanks largely to her efforts to keep up with her sister. She loves to sit and play Monopoly Junior or UNO with her sister and moms for hours. She is much more shy and reserved in crowds but has become popular in her class at school and has several good friends. She is in the young threes class three days a week at the preschool her sister attends. Although she disliked leaving her mother when she first started class at two years of age, she now wishes she could attend school every day.

Amy is large for her age. She is in the seventy-fifth to ninetieth percentiles in height, weight, and head size. She weighs more than her older sister and can share her sister's clothes. Amy has maintained her voracious appetite and loves to eat. She is physically coordinated as well. Fortunately, Amy has not suffered any asthmatic symptoms or severe bronchial infections since she came home. Of course, we immediately treat even the slightest cold or cough she experiences with every over-the-counter medicine we can find to avoid any pulmonary complications. All in all, after a harrowing start in China, Amy has proven to be a healthy, happy, well-adjusted child. Her addition to our family has made us complete. The girls are best friends as well as sisters, and we are thankful that we adopted Amy just before the Chinese government moved to make such adoptions impossible.

ADOPTIONS FROM CHINA TODAY

We have had two very positive experiences with Chinese international adoption. Unfortunately, the Chinese government has drastically changed its adoption policies in the past few years. There were two major changes. First, the CAC in China has set a quota for single-parent adoptions. Second, the Chinese government has begun requiring all adoption agencies to ensure that children are not matched into gay and lesbian homes. This has been accomplished largely through the requirement that every prospective adoptive parent sign an affidavit swearing that he or she is not engaged in nor planning to be engaged in an intimate relationship with any person of the same gender.

When we adopted both girls, Tina applied for the adoptions as a single parent, with Lee officially designated as her roommate. An unofficial "don't ask, don't tell" scenario existed. The local adoption agency was aware of the extent of our relationship, but the entire application process was based on Tina's fitness as a single parent. The question of sexual orientation was never directly asked by our International Adoption Agency or by the CAC in China. As a result, we never had to lie directly to anyone. Now we hear stories of single parents seeking adoption in China having to swear out affidavits that they are not homosexual. We never would have signed such a document. In effect, China has slammed the door on many potential caring, loving homes.

Also, in setting a quota for single-parent adoptions, the Chinese government has created what we anticipate will be a much longer waiting period for single men or women to be matched with their Chinese daughters. This will likely discourage many potential single parents altogether. The announcement of these recent policies will likely cause many single parents to disfavor China as an international adoption destination. While we do not know the total number of single-parent international adoptions from China since 1992, when the adoptions were first opened, in our two travel groups alone, thirteen out of the total thirty girls, or 43 percent, were adopted by single moms.

Of course, we feel extremely fortunate to have been able to adopt our two daughters prior to these changes. However, we are both very saddened by the loss of wonderful potential homes to which children in China will be denied access.

For any married couples who would like to adopt a healthy daughter, China should be strongly considered. The new rules require that a couple must be at least thirty years old to adopt a healthy infant, but that is one of the few restrictions. The process of adoption is truly a matter of paperwork and the home study. So long as the couple complete all paperwork appropriately, make sufficient income to support a child, and pass the criminal checks and other routine health requirements, the process guarantees that they will receive a healthy infant. There are no political uncertainties and no unexpected delays with any court processes in China. Most important, unlike in so many other foreign countries, these wonderful little Chinese girls are in the care of orphanages because they have been abandoned by their birth mothers. The parents are literally unknown. There is no possibility that the parents will claim their adoptive children one day, and an adoptive parent can rest assured that his or her child has not been bought or stolen out of an unwilling home.

The joy we have found because we adopted our daughters from China has many levels and has transformed our lives to unimaginable depths. We have been blessed not only with their presence in our family but also with the addition of our daughters' Chinese cultural heritage. We began the process of educating our daughters and ourselves about their Chinese cultural heritage by preparing adoption books for each of them. These books explain and describe how we chose to adopt, when we learned who our daughters would be, and about our trips to China to bring our daughters home, and they include maps, pictures, and histories of the provinces and cities of our daughters' births. We read these books and watch our travel videos from our trips to China whenever the girls request them, which is often.

We have also attended many events at the local Chinese cultural center, which is part of the Chinese community that has settled in our city. Lia's preschool teacher is Chinese and an active participant in programs at this cultural center. We have learned of and attended several events through our connection with her. She has also informed us that she teaches Chinese, but she does not want to teach us while Lia is still her student at the preschool. We hope to have her teach us Chinese beginning this summer. We listen to Chinese music and try to learn Chinese songs as a family. Lia and Amy show great affinity for this endeavor. Amy loves to sing her Chinese songs, and we look up Chinese words in our dictionary at Lia's constant insistence. We also have Chinese computer programs to help teach us Chinese. We regularly eat Chinese food and delight in "dim sum" brunch at a local Chinese restaurant. We have decorated our house with art that we brought back from China. We hope by doing all of this we can help our daughters learn how they can integrate their Chinese and American cultures into their lives.

Finally, we are members of a large local chapter of Families with Children from China. This group arranges or attends many cultural and social events, including Chinese New Year and Autumn Moon celebrations, dragon dances, Chinese dance festivals, nature hikes, and play dates. Participation in this group has allowed us to provide our family with exposure to events of cultural significance for Chinese people and to form a new cultural subgroup of families with adopted Chinese children. Our Chinese-American daughters will one day be a group of women possessed of their own special heritage. It is impossible for us to know or imagine the future that will be created by this remarkable group of women brought out of China to America as babies. We believe that humanity can only benefit from the loving diversity embodied in these Chinese-American daughters with whom we have created our families.

Chapter 7

From One Wondrous Second to Countless Memorable Moments: Adventures in Adoption

Pamela Diane Dunne

It lasted but a second, but it was a second I will never forget— a second that erased any small doubts I may have had about the adoption process, a second that confirmed the wisdom of my decision to adopt, a second that transformed my hopes and dreams and fears into pure visceral, guttural joy, a second that immediately brought tears to my eyes then, and even now as I relive it. It was the second when I kissed my infant daughter for the first time. I had just seen her for the first time a few hours earlier, but this was our first time alone together. She bumped her head against her crib, not particularly hard, not hard enough to cause her to cry, but hard enough for my natural maternal instinct to respond immediately with a kiss to her head. And that is when it happened, the second that I will never forget, the second that gives me goose bumps even now. For it was in that second that I realized immediately, instinctively, intuitively, to my surprise, that she had never been kissed. I cannot tell you exactly how or why I knew, but I did. And as I looked into her wide, saucerlike eyes and saw in them her mixture of surprise and confusion, but mostly happiness and comfort, the tears welling up in my own eyes reflected the flood of feelings her reaction to my kiss elicited in me. It was all of a second, but in that second I felt a sense of pure joy that has stayed with me like no other, and despite all the many seconds and hours and days of pure joy that my two adopted children have brought me in the seven years since then, the beauty of adoption will always be captured best for me in that one wondrous second.

The road which led me to that memorable second was a winding one, particularly in light of the fact that I already was a single parent of four biological children (from a former marriage) who were at the time ages ten years through adulthood. Two children lived with me in Malibu, California, one attended college away from home, and the other lived in her own apartment. Today, Sami (my oldest daughter) works as an interior designer, actress, and makeup artist. Krista completed her BA in poetry and playwriting at the University of California, Santa Cruz, and assists in managing a new business while continuing to write. Reese recently completed his BA at the University of California, Santa Cruz, in digital film and will be living and working in New Zealand for a year. Karina is a college sophomore majoring in interior design/photography and works as a professional model/actress. I began the adoption process in 1993 and completed my first adoption in 1995. After earning two PhDs (one in theater and the other in clinical psychology), I continue to juggle hats as a professor of theater arts and dance at California State University, Los Angeles, and director of the Drama Therapy Institute of Los Angeles.

ADOPTION WONDERINGS

Contemplating dreams and possibilities, a familiar posture to me, I began thinking about adopting two orphan children (a boy and a girl) from different cultures. I chose not to consider an adoption in the United States because my heart beat for the children in foreign countries who were being raised in orphanages (to be eligible for foreign adoption, a child must be abandoned). While some individuals at my place in the life cycle (middle age) look forward to their children growing up (freeing up their time and energies), I knew within every fiber of my being that I wanted to continue my child rearing for the next twenty years. I really missed little children. Some friends and family members questioned why I wanted to continue raising children when my life would soon be free of these responsibilities. I believe that my special gifts lie in the area of nurturing parent/teacher and in celebrating play, creativity, and discovery. As I am very committed to my biological children, we engaged in long discussions about this topic, and my passions became known. My teenage children, very absorbed in their own lives, failed to understand the significance of this to me (although they tried).

I began contemplating the effect that adoption would have on my family, future, time, profession, and other aspects of my life. Reviewing my most important moments in life—the birth of my son (three months early), Sami saying "hi" when she was three months old, my special New York trips with Krista to experience live theater, and Karina's memorable letter to me during her one-year exchange program in Sweden—I discovered all were child related. I also remember milestones in my professional life—promotion to professor, author of eight books, president of National Association of Drama Therapy, and leader of four drama therapy workshops in Kuwait. While these achievements enriched my life, moments with my children clearly ranked on top. Reflecting on how my children would adapt to a new sibling, I truly believed that they all possessed such big hearts, sensitivity, and depth that they would find a way to open themselves to a new little one. Adoption offered opportunities for our family to grow outside of the known, to become less self-centered, and to share our abundant lives with a little child. Offering a new future and hope for a child struck me as an incredible opportunity. I knew that as much as I gave to a child, my returns would be hundredfold. A Malibu family who had adopted twenty-eight children from various parts of the world inspired me, and I began asking questions, researching adoptions in foreign countries, attending adoption conferences, joining adoption groups, and reading many books. Thus this incredible and rewarding journey began.

ADOPTION DISAPPOINTMENTS

Looking down this road, little did I realize the extensive time, major disappointments, and turns in the way; however, guided by my passions and determination, I could visualize a successful outcome. I was older than the preferred age (middle age eliminated many possibilities), single (married couples preferred), not childless (childless couples preferred), with limited financial resources ($20,000 required for adoption costs), and on and on. I began working with a lawyer in Alaska who was handling adoptions in Moscow (he charged a reasonable fee) and, after a year of completing a home study with the social worker at Vista Del Mar and the appropriate paperwork, I made a trip to Russia, visited a medical facility, and bonded with a beautiful little baby girl who was available for adoption. This international adoption involved one attorney and a hired agent working with that attorney in Moscow. After spending two days with this sweet child, whom I called Kayla, an agent hired by my lawyer told me to go home and that I would be returning to Moscow in four to six months pending completion of the paperwork. Sadly, I took Kayla on a stroll the last day, prayed that God would keep her safe, took pictures, left medical supplies and clothing (gifts for the facility), and boarded the plane for home. Agonizing months went by, and finally a year of long phone calls, additional paperwork, and delays passed with my family on edge awaiting this event. My lawyer regretfully informed me that adoption laws in Russia had changed (one of the major risks in international adoption is the changeability of laws and regulations with no notice), and that Kayla had been taken away from me and given to a young couple. Due to my age, single status, and the fact that I had other children, the new adoption law rendered me ineligible. Depressed about this for weeks, I placed Kayla's pictures in a special scrapbook, searched for a way to find closure, and prayed for God's blessing on her life. A friend of mine suggested I try China, a much smoother road with less strict laws and a history of success stories.

THE ARRIVAL OF ZOË

With hope for the future, I contacted U.S. Asian Affairs (a small, recommended agency), taking another six months to prepare paperwork for China. This could not have gone more smoothly; Norman Niu (director of U.S. Asian Affairs) handled everything with sensitivity and professionalism (different from my failed experience in Russia). About six months into the process, Norman excitedly called me about a two-month-old baby girl who had been brought to the orphanage in Sanshui, informing me that if I chose her, I would leave for China in two to three months. My heart raced at the anticipation of a dream coming true, and I asked about her medical records. In foreign adoptions medical records from third world countries are often unreliable and brief. I received the following medical information about Zoë (my name for her):

Sex: F
Age: 2 months
Residence: Welfare Institution
Height: 60 cm (24 inches)
Weight: 5.8 kg (approximately 10 lb)
Skin, thyroid gland, limbs, joints, lymph, and spine: normal
Eyes, ears, nose, throat, and mouth: normal
Development and nutrition: medium
Mental and nervous system: normal
Lungs and respiratory tract: normal
Heart and blood vessels: normal
Liver and spleen: normal
HbsAg: negative
Result: healthy
Date of exam: January 11, 1996

My family physician reviewed this information and found no obvious red flags. I decided to go ahead and immediately called Norman with my approval and arranged to provide funds for a special caretaker for my child. Excitement spread as my other family members began anticipating the arrival of this little girl. We agreed as a family to call her Zoë Arianna (Zoë was my daughter Krista's favorite name, and we all liked Arianna, too). The law required that the baby be a minimum of three months of age before leaving China. During this waiting period, U.S. Asian Affairs prepared many of the documents that I needed to proceed which were notarized and sent ahead. Agents of U.S. Asian Affairs in China handled additional documents. I invited Karina (twelve years of age at that time) to come with me, and in March 1996 we boarded a plane with Norman Niu and ten other individuals who were adopting (couples and singles). We landed in Hong Kong to rest up and then went on to southern China to Guangzhou. A few days later, the other adoptive parents (and some children), Karina, and I boarded a charted bus that took us to the orphanage. It took about an hour to get from Guangzhou in Sunshui.

Waiting in a small room of this large orphanage, we experienced an atmosphere of anticipation, nervousness, and excitement. The first child to be adopted celebrated her first birthday that day and we all sang "Happy Birthday" as her adoptive mom (a single parent with a Chinese daughter) eagerly took her. Then a childless couple who had tried unsuccessfully for fifteen years to bear children received their little girl. I still remember their incredibly happy faces as they held their little girl for the first time. We all cried with them as flashing cameras filled the room. Then a second couple that had one son received their little girl. The little boy (who was about six) beamed as he saw his new sister. Then it was our turn. Karina stood by the outside door, as she wanted to be the first to see Zoë. Then I saw the face of a little baby peering out from a blanket covering her head, looking around the room curiously. Dressed in layers of clothes and wrapped in several blankets, she looked like a chubby bear cub. Karina undressed Zoë (four months of age) and put her in a cute red ladybug outfit, and one of the couples gave us a little pink hat to go with it. Adorable with her chubby cheeks, she enjoyed moving her legs and arms, which had been all bound up.

In a journal entry of March 25, 1996 (date of receiving Zoë), I wrote:

> Zoë, when I adopted you and saw you for the first time, you were brought to me and you turned your head to look at everyone and you smiled. You were dressed in many layers of clothes and it was difficult for you to move. Your sister Karina dressed you in a new ladybug one-piece outfit and a couple that had come on the trip with us gave you a cute pink hat. You could move your head from side to side, almost roll on your side, and could not sit up unless someone was holding you.

When all the families received their children, we celebrated with a catered lunch at the orphanage. Leaving gifts for the orphanage, we boarded the bus with our babies and went back to the White Swan Hotel, where a trained staff greeted us, eager to help. Karina and I could not get to the phone fast enough to call home, and then all the questions came: "How big is she?" "Is she healthy?" "What did she do when she first saw you?" and so on. In the next two fantastic weeks while the final paperwork, immigration forms, and passports were being prepared, daily sight-seeing trips, luncheons, and dinners were planned with all the families and babies. All scheduled meetings with government officials and immigration were handled by a staff member of U.S. Asian Affairs and the prospective parents. Celebrating meals at large round tables in restaurants in Guangzhou, all of us bonded with one another while eating, talking, and enjoying the in-

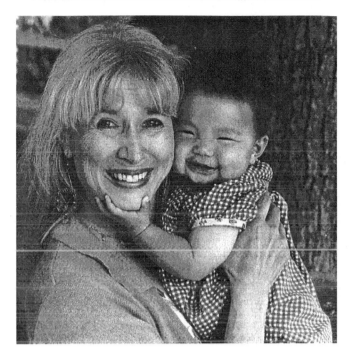

Pam and Zoë

credible sights of China. Because of my experience with children, I became the resident expert—a role I really enjoyed. Finally our last day in Guangzhou arrived; we gathered for an incredible farewell party and dinner at a gourmet restaurant. It was the perfect conclusion to celebrate what would change our lives forever. Everything had proceeded exactly as planned, and there were no hidden costs or extended overseas stays necessary. Upon arriving home, Zoë became fully adjusted to her new surroundings in about a month (she was a very easy and patient baby). To bring in the larger support structure of friends and extended family, a birth announcement heralding the arrival of Zoë brought everyone together for a celebration of dinner, cake, and gifts. Zoë quickly discovered the joy of opening presents, and this process appeared to be as much fun as the actual product received. With this ritual, Zoë (especially cute with her fat little cheeks) officially took on her new role as a family member, and the first part of my dream came true.

THE ARRIVAL OF ZACHARY

A year later my son Reese (age eighteen) and I boarded a plane to Cambodia, working with Maine Adoption Service (a recommended agency), Seattle Adoption Agency (an intermediary), and Lauryn Galindo (an agent working for Seattle Adoption Agency living in Cambodia), to receive a Cambodian baby boy. Boys were not available in China, so I decided to try Vietnam, putting my name on a waiting list. One day I received a call from the director of Maine Adoption Service, asking me if I could go in the next month to Cambodia and saying that there were some baby boys available in a small orphanage. One of them she described from his medical records as a happy, affectionate baby with excellent motor skills. "That sounds like the one. Can you keep him safe for me until I can get there?" I chose the name Zachary (going so well with Zoë) and anticipated the arrival of a promised photograph. When it arrived, I put little Zachary's picture in the middle of a family collage and sent it out on all our Christmas cards.

Before leaving for Cambodia, I wrote a letter to Suy Sem, the Cambodian secretary of state, stating my intention to adopt:

October 21, 1996

Honorable Sir:

I am writing this letter to introduce myself to you. I am a professor at California State University and specialize in helping children, teens, and families. I work with children in both therapy and education and have helped children with emotional and educational problems for over fifteen years. I care very much for children and feel that I can offer a Cambodian child a family with love and resources to grow and develop. I want to adopt a Cambodian child because I love children, and raising children has been one of the most wonderful and rewarding experiences in my life. Upon completion of the adoption, the child will take on my family name and have full inheritance rights upon my death. The child will have the opportunity for higher education and will not be abused or abandoned. I will provide love and nurturing and make sure that my child will be exposed to the values and culture of the Cambodian people.

I wanted to take Reese to Cambodia, as he had hoped for years for a brother. Between October and December 1996, I completed some of the necessary paperwork, which needed to be notarized. In January 1997, I received a note from Cambodia from Lauryn (excerpted here):

Aloha from Cambodia.

I know that for many of you this will be your first visit to a third world country. It will be helpful for you to read back issues of *National Geographic* to see pictures of Cambodia and to speak with adoptive parents who have traveled there. I ask for your patience and to trust me to handle any unusual circumstances. Even during the armed conflict, I got all "my kids" to safety with completed visas. At the same time that I am finalizing your child's adoption and facilitating a timely departure, I am frequently meeting with dignitaries trying to keep the program running. Cambodians are very protective of the orphans of their nation. Try to remain flexible, know that EVERY adoptive family that I have submitted to the Cambodian government has been approved and has left the country with their child or I have personally escorted the child to the parents. Enjoy your experience. The Khmer are a warm, friendly people with a rich heritage. Soak it up so you can tell your child about their birthplace. Take a car around the city, visit the marketplaces, buy jewels (rubies and sapphires are very reasonable), see the Royal Palace and the Silver Pagoda, and go to Mekong Island to see traditional arts and crafts. Speak with the people and you will discover that their stories are all heartbreaking. Return home with your precious child and a renewed appreciation for the blessing we take for granted. Remember you are all my heroes coming to rescue the orphans from an uncertain future.

Much Love,
Lauryn Galindo

In January 1997, Reese and I left for Cambodia. Unlike my experience in China, the Cambodian trip involved the individual parent going over (not as part of a group), and no structured activities, events, or meals were planned. Each family, upon arrival in Cambodia, heard from Lauryn, who arranged a driver (hired for a fee). About one hour after arriving in Phnom Penh, I received a phone call saying that our driver would be picking us up to take us to the orphanage. We hurriedly got everything together, with our excitement-generated adrenaline rush keeping us going even though we were very tired and suffering from jet lag. Our driver took us just out of town on a small dirt road with goats and cows blocking the roadway. Finally we arrived at a small orphanage (a tentlike structure with open sides), where two lovely Cambodian women greeted us warmly. Children were resting on small grass mats on the floor or being rocked to sleep in large hammocks. The caretaker whom I had arranged to care for my child prior to arrival handed Zachary to me for the first time. No one spoke any English at the orphanage, so our driver handled all the translation. We learned that Zachary loved a fish soup (indigenous to Cambodia), and we saw as he moved on the floor that he had highly developed motor skills, unlike the Chinese babies who were confined in cribs and wrapped tightly in blankets. Cambodian babies crawled freely on a wooden floor and experienced little confinement. Older Cambodian women were selling beautiful cloths at the orphanage, and we bought some to take home. We took little Zachary back to our hotel room (in culture shock and jet-lagged), armed with formula brought from the United States and this special fish soup, and took a long nap. Later we met with Lauryn to complete paperwork, and then our driver took us around the city to historical sights, markets, and temples while we took lots of pictures and continued to get acquainted with Zachary.

A few days later we met some other families who had just arrived, and together we hired drivers to take us to the beach. (Lauryn operated another part of the orphanage there, a four-hour trip away, and she invited us all to come.) We spent some time in hammocks on the beach, had dinner, and then both Reese and I became very sick (food poisoning, we believe). After throwing up for hours, I finally got better, but Reese continued to get worse, developing a fever. In the middle of the night, I frantically called Lauryn, who came to pick us up and arranged to meet a doctor at the hospital. They put Reese on a stretcher outside the entrance of the hospital (space not available in the hospital) and, to give him some fluids, suspended an IV from a wall crawling with insects. This outside area, much cleaner and more sanitary than the inside area, certainly failed to meet the lowest stan-

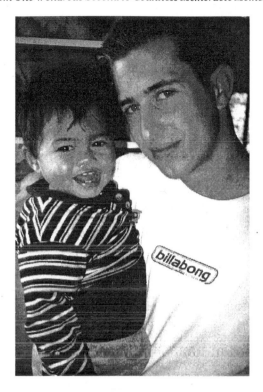

Zachary and Reese

dards of care and sanitation in the United States. Reese continued to throw up despite medication; he felt absolutely miserable. I sang songs to him, held his hand, and prayed. Finally, when morning came, Reese's vomiting lessened and his fever broke. Totally exhausted, on our way back to the United States, we arranged for an overnight room in Thailand and slept. We were in Phnom Penh about a week and then returned to Malibu with Zachary.

Zachary arrived one year after Zoë, and again my older children were surprised, mainly that this second adoption had happened so soon. A smoother adjustment to Zachary (paved by Zoë's earlier entrance) occurred as the family, already used to crying at night, bottles, playpens, and other baby things, adapted quickly. All the little things that babies bring became a part of the everyday existence of the family. In the midst of all the girls (four sisters) and one older brother, a

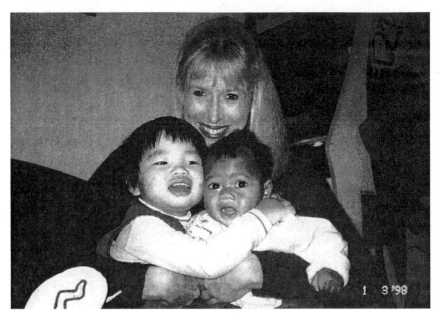

Zoë, Zachary, and Pam

little boy in the family became a major event. Sleeping through the night and adapting so well to things, Zachary made his entrance to America quite smoothly.

ZOË AND ZACHARY THEN AND TODAY

Zoë Arianna, a sweet, sensitive child, lacked opportunities to develop her motor skills due to being wrapped all the time and confined to a crib prior to adoption. Developmentally, except for motor skills, she responded age appropriately, and her weight and height were within the normal range. All her medical tests in the United States came back normal, and within her first week in this country she began getting her infant inoculations. Filled with boundless curiosity, easy to care for, and adaptable, Zoë quickly captured the hearts of the entire family. Once she had opportunities to crawl, sit, and move, her motor skills developed. She began sleeping through the night and bonding with family members.

Zoë's Development

Today, Zoë excels in gymnastics and swimming and has pride in her abilities on the trampoline and in the swimming pool. Having a wonderful sense of rhythm, she enjoys dancing (sensing the beat and improvising steps), singing, and drama (acting out stories and seeing plays). Her eagerness to learn and conscientious attitude toward homework and other tasks are evident in school (she is in the first grade). Learning Chinese and Spanish quickly, she prides herself on knowing how to count and engage in simple conversation. In social settings, her sense of loyalty to friends results in positive relationships. Other family members describe her as intelligent, creative, curious, competitive, loyal, talkative, sensitive, affectionate, and loving.

I observed that, as a young child, Zoë needed to gain confidence in herself (appreciating talents and abilities). This was accomplished through structure, repetition, and practice of tasks. For example, in learning to ride a bike, Zoë required more time than Zachary to feel comfortable. Zachary began riding a two-wheeler right away; he never gave up when he was first learning. Zoë, on the other hand, had the tendency to be critical of herself when she failed to do something to her satisfaction. Recognition, praise, and appreciation of Zoë's positive qualities and efforts helped her. Accepting criticism, another very difficult task for Zoë (even if the criticism was well meaning and gentle), sometimes resulted in her overreacting by crying profusely or saying, "You don't like me." Separation created much anxiety, perhaps triggered by fear of abandonment. Trying to be sensitive to Zoë's needs, I adjusted my work schedule, taking Zoë with me to out-of-town conventions and spending as much time as I could with her. This brought back many happy memories of years gone by when I had taken my four older children with me to conventions. Separation continued to be a problem through age five, although Zoë improved significantly as she became more secure, sure of herself, and confident. As for discipline, I tried to be very gentle (especially in the tone of my voice) and assuring, but firm. At age six, Zoë began showing more confidence in her abilities, perhaps due in part to her special talents in gymnastics and swimming, positive feedback, and popularity in her school class. Zoë's teacher said of her, "Everybody likes Zoë, all the girls and the boys. She is one of the most popular children in the class." Problematic behaviors with respect to separation and extreme sensitivity began subsiding and were replaced by the more positive and adaptive behaviors of self-confidence, reasonability, and enhanced self-control.

Zachary's Development

Zachary Osar, as an infant, slept on a floor mat, crawled and moved much of the day, and developed advanced motor skills for his age. A friendly, happy child, Zachary won the hearts of the family with his engaging smile and large dark eyes. His medical tests as an infant came back basically normal, although he experienced some ongoing problems with congestion/breathing, which today have resulted in athletic asthma. Developmentally and physically on track, Zachary began showing spurts of growth and weight gain. Zachary's easygoing, calm personality helped him adjust to new situations without experiencing stress. Although he encountered some difficulty with potty training, Zachary improved with this when he started preschool. A very friendly child, Zachary forms social relationships easily and eagerly approaches new situations. Separation issues were not a major problem, and he easily plays at the homes of his new friends, adjusts to different baby-sitters, and handles other changes without much difficulty. Zachary and Zoë adapted very quickly to each other, bonding, becoming very close, and not wanting to be separated from each other, notwithstanding occasional sibling rivalry. Zachary will enter kindergarten at age five. He loves "Thomas the Tank Engine," bike and scooter riding, gymnastics, swimming, rock climbing, soccer, and T-ball. A very bright child, Zachary learns very quickly and wants to know everything that Zoë knows, often wanting to complete the same homework she has, and he has also been learning Chinese and Spanish. They do everything together and miss each other greatly when they are apart, greeting each other with a big hug and "I love you." Family members describe Zachary as easygoing, funny, playful, sweet, affectionate, sensitive, shy, smart, and adventurous.

Changing Family Dynamics

Zoë and Zachary became sister and brother, respectively, to four older siblings who all had different views about adoption. Three were teenagers/preteens highly involved in their own lives (concerned that something would be taken away from them due to new responsibilities toward the little ones), and one was a single working woman on her own. However, Zoë and Zachary quickly endeared themselves to the entire family, winning their hearts and love. The dynamic of older siblings assists in creating a strong support structure and invites these older siblings to become role models. Family Sunday brunch, an important ritual, took on new meaning. The older ones, because of the large age difference, feel no competition with the little ones and genuinely enjoy taking them on activities (movies, overnight). Grandparents Millie and Vern Peterson (my mom and dad), although they did not initially understand my reasons for adoption, were nonetheless supportive, becoming very proud grandparents.

Extended Support

Not long after adopting Zachary, I became very close to Jonathan, a dear friend. Jonathan loved kids and bonded with the children very easily by showing them magic tricks the first day he met them (magic was a hobby for him). Little Zachary began saying "matra" for magic whenever he saw Jonathan. Jonathan, by establishing a supportive, loving relationship with the children, was assisting in constructing the building blocks of love and trust. This also expanded the loving support and honored the children.

MY ADOPTION INSIGHTS

Although I would not want to repeat what happened in Russia with losing Kayla, without any reservation I would repeat the adoption experience, which remains one of the most important, significant, and positive decisions of my life. This decision helped me to grow in compassion, patience, and trust of God. My growth as a person through this experience resulted in a depth and maturity not present before. After I visited various developing countries and observed the extensive poverty, lack of sophisticated medical facilities and staff, lack of resources, and difficulty in daily existence, my worldview changed significantly. Compassion, acceptance, and respect for different religious, cultural, and racial groups increased. Gaining empathy, understanding, and a love for others through these experiences continues to impact my life profoundly.

Increased compassion for others affects my work in group homes as a psychologist/drama therapist. I witness daily the hurt, anger, and disillusionment of abandoned children. Crying out for love, these teens act out, show rage, assume attitudes, drop out of school, and, in any other way they can, try to get attention. Underneath their anger are hurt and the deep desire for togetherness, a yearning for a family and for someone to love them. In group homes with younger children, I test babies (some with medical or neurological problems) who, again, through no fault of their own, live in institutions with not enough caregivers to provide for the needs of all who require their time and love. With so many homeless children not experiencing the joy of a family and suffering the effects of institutionalism, I worry for the future of a world that has lost the stability of the family. I only hope that more families, singles, and other persons with a desire to adopt will reach out to homeless children of all ages throughout the world and bring them into their lives.

Adoption Pitfalls

Doing more in-depth research into foreign adoption could possibly have helped me avoid the pitfalls I encountered in Moscow. Working with a lawyer, not an established agency, constituted a more risky situation. Although his intentions were honest, this lawyer was not fully prepared to deal with all the brick walls and conflicts encountered, whereas an agency with a proven track record may have known how to circumvent these problems. I chose a lawyer rather than an agency because of the prohibitive agency costs (around $20,000 and above), and my limited funds prevented me from pursuing a large agency. Talking to other adoptive parents (getting references) and making extensive phone calls finally resulted in the discovery of the two least expensive but reliable agencies, moving the adoption process smoothly and efficiently to its conclusion: the adoptions of Zoë and Zachary.

After what I had been through in Russia, my trip to China felt like a fairy tale come true. Maine Adoption Service worked with the Seattle Adoption Agency and Lauryn Galindo in Cambodia, and this resulted in dealings with many different people, organizations, and multiple layers of paperwork. Lauryn Galindo, the only contact person in Cambodia, worked single-handedly raising money for needy children, taking homeless children on all kinds of special trips and events, and raising funds to help with poverty. A focus on more structured events (e.g., dinners, field trips) would have added significantly to my experience in Cambodia, but I recognize that Lauryn, already overworked and overextended, could not do more. Most adoptive parents arriving in Cambodia stayed only a few days, but I wanted to experience Cambodia and bring back special remembrances of the country to keep for Zachary. My son and I stayed a week, as we wanted to be able to see some of the country, to experience the people, customs, and culture.

Honoring My Children's Cultural Heritage

Keeping children in touch with their cultural heritage allows them to experience the dignity and respect that their culture deserves. Zoë and Zachary show pride in being Chinese and Cambodian, respectively, as well as pride in being American. Learning Chinese brings excitement to Zoë, who feels proud to learn the language of her native country. Zoë celebrates Chinese New Year, attends reunions with Chinese adoptive parents, and learns songs and stories from China, all contributing to her pride and cultural heritage. I found a support group in Los Angeles for families who have adopted Cambodian children that offers opportunities to attend birthdays, reunions, Cambodian New Year celebrations, and other special events. Experiencing Chinese and Cambodian food has given each child exposure to that aspect of his or her country. Our bringing back important cultural artifacts, pictures, musical instruments, cloth, and other items from both Cambodia and China has also served to put the children in touch with their culture.

Assessing Risk

One of my best life decisions was to adopt a child. Having raised and nurtured four biological children, I observe no difference in my commitment, love, and bonding with my precious adopted children. I feel especially privileged to be able to give Zoë and Zachary a new abundant life filled with love, support, opportunities, and challenges. I can honestly say that doubts about adoption were not a part of my thinking. High on my list of "must haves," outranking anything else, was adopting a healthy child. Because of work and personal responsibility for my other children, no available time for a special needs child existed in my life; however, foreign adoption, in particular, leaves many unanswered questions about issues of health. Due to the limited medical records and lack of information on the child's history, definite risks exist that a child may carry certain undiagnosed medical conditions or psychological problems. I consider myself very fortunate that Zoë and Zachary came to me reasonably nourished, healthy, and with no medical problems, as confirmed by their first exams in the United States.

REFLECTIONS TODAY

As I began driving back with Zoë from Mother/Daughter Camp (sponsored by Forest Home Christian Center), a special weekend for mothers and daughters, I reviewed in my mind the events of that weekend. I fondly reflected on how Zoë's outgoing, alive, and vibrant personality was received by people in the camp (inviting comments such as, "She's certainly not shy") and on her deep affection and love for her family. I thought back to when I first saw Zoë as a baby (looking curiously around the room) and then to Zoë now—confident, assertive, creative, and endearing with her sweet sensitivity. She had been looking forward to this weekend for a year and had been determined to experience every moment of it to the fullest, from singing praises to God to swimming, tetherball, miniature golf, karaoke, and roasting marshmallows. I remembered how Zachary hugged me as I left and whispered in my ear, "I love you," and I assured him he would be going to a mother/son weekend soon. I also thought about similar trips that I had made with my adult children which offered great bonding and enriching experiences, and now history was repeating itself. My thoughts compelled me to realize how much I love spending time with my grown up-children as well. We go to the theater, the fruit market, films, dinner, plays, and special outings in the park and make meals together (our favorite is Sunday brunch). My older children are my favorite people with whom I talk, spend time, and share. Upon arriving home I spotted Zachary and Jonathan on the upstairs balcony, looking like twins of a sort, both dressed in jeans and T-shirts with caps pulled down. I had missed them both so much. We could not get to each other fast enough to have a "group hug" (a family tradition). In the moment of that warm hug and exchange of

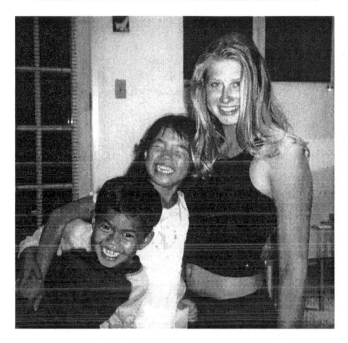

Zachary, Zoë, and Karina

the words "I love you," I silently thanked God for giving me Zoë and Zachary who continue to bless and bring joy in my life every day. From that joyous second when I first kissed Zoë's head, through the countless moments of pleasure and love since, my heart has been filled with gratitude for the gifts that adoption has given me.

ADDENDUM BY KARINA BARRAGAR

When I was ten years old my mother said that she wanted to have another child and nothing would stand in her way. My mother wanted to adopt a child, but all of my siblings and I were against her decision, not because it was adoption, but because she wanted another child. Even though all of us were against her proposal, she went ahead with her decision.

Two years later, my mom and I were on our way to China to adopt my little sister, Zoë. I was worried at first, thinking that she would have some defect or a major health problem, but Mom assured me that there was nothing to worry about, because she was going to be a part of the family and why would that even be relevant. In China, other singles and couples who were also adopting children surrounded my mother and me. Everyone's eyes were filled with wonderment and, sharing these feelings, we all grew very close together as a group and even as a family. All of us were waiting patiently for the day when we would go as a group on a chartered bus to the orphanage in Sansui and see our new children. When we arrived at the orphanage, my heart was beating very fast. I knew that soon I would be meeting my new little sister. That day still seems to have been the longest day of my life. Soon enough, little girls were brought out one by one, all of us waiting patiently to receive ours. Finally they called my mother's name and I ran outside so I could be the first to see her, my little sister. Tears came to my eyes when I saw her, and upon seeing my mother carry her daughter for the first time.

Now that I am eighteen, I realize that there was never a thought in my mind about regretting my mom's decision. I do feel bad for feeling the way I did when my mother told me that she wanted another child. Even though I am not the youngest anymore, I now have a beautiful, intelligent sister of whom I am so proud. Sometimes I feel as if she is my child because I was there in the beginning, and I will always be there for her, but I guess that is just the role of a big sister.

ADDENDUM BY REESE BARRAGAR

Overall it has been an amazing experience with Zack, from the time I traveled to Cambodia with my mother to pick him up to the present. Zack is a loving, exciting, and warm child who has given me an opportunity to play the role of an older brother. Just a couple of months ago I taught him how to ride his bike without training wheels (which he picked up really quickly, especially for a four-year-old).

When my mother and I first saw Zack on a small grass mat in the Cambodian orphanage, I was appalled by the living conditions of these poor children but felt better when I understood what my mother and the several others there were doing—providing these children with love and care in a healthier environment for them to grow up in.

The way I feel about Zack and Zoë is the same way I feel toward my other siblings. Even though Zack and Zoë look nothing like anyone in our family, they still know and understand (to a certain degree) who their family is and who their big brother is. Part of the adoptive process is letting the child know who the family is, no matter what skin color or other external features may be different. I feel that Zack and Zoë both acknowledge that their appearances are different from ours but understand that we are their family despite the differences.

Overall, I feel that having an adopted brother and sister is just like having a normal sibling. The advantages of adopting are extraordinary. Just the realization that one is providing a beneficial environment for a child with no family is amazing. Zack and Zoë are two beautiful young children who have a bright future ahead of them, and being a part of their lives has been a remarkable experience in itself.

ADDENDUM BY SAMANTHA BARRAGAR

Two children sit on a concrete step, arms interwoven, surrounded by a blanket of upturned leaves. Looking at them with heads close together and smiles of cheerful mischief on their faces, one would never know that this boy and girl were not biological siblings—as one seems to complete the other. As my own smile begins in return, I realize that I cannot imagine now what life would be like without them.

Zoë came first, the last and best present on that forthcoming Christmas day—wide eyed and silent, taking in everything. My family was nervous and excited at the same time. How would this new member of our family affect our lives? I was in my midtwenties—could I really be a sister to someone three months old who could easily be my daughter? All of us had our own secret apprehensions. But as her eyes met mine for the first time, these apprehensions seemed to disappear and were replaced by a strong desire to shower this little child with as much love as I could possibly give.

As Zoë began to grow, my mother started having thoughts of a second adoption—this way, Zoë could have a little brother or sister to grow up with, as all of us were so much older. She spent countless hours searching and waiting until finally the opportunity arose. A little boy in Cambodia needed a home, so off she went, not letting anything stand in her way. In what seemed like moments, Zachary arrived, filled with energy and a sporting a quizzical smile.

Today Zach and Zoë are an inseparable pair. My sister and my boyfriend and I love to have slumber parties and rent cartoons, filling the house with popcorn, candy wrappers, and laughter. All of the best experiences we had as children ourselves we want to pass on in all their glory: flying a kite, roller-coaster rides, the excitement of a new toy, ice skates, dress up, tea parties, hide-and-seek. When any of us come to visit, we can hear our names being joyfully called out as two small bundles of energy come running up to us, arms outstretched.

Zach and Zoë are the greatest gifts our family could have ever received. I look forward to traveling with them someday back to China and Cambodia, so they can experience the beautiful heritage that they descended from and learn about their native countries. I imagine them in high school, graduating college, getting married, and having families of their own. I anticipate the amazing things they will do and the incredible people they will become. Two children sit on a concrete step, surrounded by love, hope, family, and future— a future of which we are all honored to be a part.

ADDENDUM BY KRISTA BARRAGAR

I thought about beginning this with a story about Zach and Zoë. There are so many snippets and moments in which I could describe my sister and brother: how Zoë continues to be silently jealous that Zach can ride a bike without training wheels, while she stops movement by dragging her heels, or how the two of them surprised us one morning by coloring all four of their bedroom walls with crayon doodles and variations on the letter Z, or when they swing dance with each other to emulate our mom's first love, or how Zoë's crooked-teeth smile mirrors a grin on another, and how Zach's big brown eyes will always brighten even a grumpy person's bad day.

I thought about how I could address the subject of this book, relating it to Zoë being Chinese and Zach being Cambodian. With Zoë's long silky black hair and Zach's coarse shaggy 'do, with their shades and facial features, I am concerned about the reactions they may receive based upon others' prejudice and reflected in looks flashed at them, in the cartoons that they watch on Saturday mornings, or inside their very own school classrooms. Part of their identity is so vastly different from our blonde hair and white skin, and a world with overt criticism and racism will, without a doubt, plague them in varying degrees throughout their lives.

The thing is, this book has to do with adoption and what we think of our adopted siblings, daughters or sons, cousins or nieces. What are our experiences? What do we want to share? So, I guess I want to say simply that I think of them as two energetic, caring, thoughtful, and usually messy little people who are just as much a part of me as I am a part of them. We are a unit, a whole, a circle, full. They are, and will always be, a constant example of a kind of luminosity that I rarely find in people, but that envelops Zoë and Zach like an embrace you never want to release.

ADDENDUM BY MILDRED PETERSON

When our daughter, Pam, adopted Zoë and Zachary, my husband, Vern, was still alive. I knew that Pam wanted more kids and I was supportive of her getting them, but even so, I had never experienced adoption before and I did not expect to like them so much. Zoë is brilliant. She has a genius mind. Zachary is very lovable. Anybody would like him. They are amazing and exceptional children. For us, there is no difference between them and our other grandchildren.

Some of my happiest memories of my husband, Vern, involve Zoë and Zachary. When Pam adopted the children, Vern and I had recently moved to Los Angeles and were living five minutes away from Pam's condo in Malibu. Vern was very proud of the children and where they were from and agreed with me that they were exceptionally smart. He often referred to Zoë as "my little China girl."

Vern died in 1999, when Zachary was not quite two and Zoë was three and a half. The children used to spend time at our condo and always looked forward to visiting us there. Toward the end, when Vern had some serious health problems and was bedridden much of the time, one of my favorite memories is of Zoë showing Vern how she had learned to swing dance. Vern had always loved dancing (just like our daughter, Pam) and he was especially touched by Zoë's little dance, and the smile on his face from that joyous moment persisted throughout the day.

We could not have better grandchildren!

Chapter 8

Welcome Home—Liv, Kim, and Love

Marianne Cederblad

I am at present sixty-seven years old and retired from my position as a professor of child and adolescent psychiatry at the University of Lund. I am Caucasian, born in Sweden by Swedish parents. I was married for some years without having any children. I adopted my three children after being divorced for several years. I worked as a child psychiatrist at different university clinics in Sweden and was appointed professor first at Umeå University in the far north of Sweden and then at Lund in the southernmost part of the country.

I have always been interested in the situation of children in different cultures. My doctoral thesis was an epidemiological study on Sudanese Arab children outside Khartoum, Sudan, where I worked as a psychiatrist for one year. I have also done research in Ethiopia, Thailand, and Iraqi Kurdistan. I have worked with humanitarian aid groups in the form of training programs for professionals in child psychiatry, teaching family therapy in Bulgaria; for staff at orphanages in Ethiopia; and for social workers and physicians working in trauma centers for children and adolescents with post-traumatic stress disorder (PTSD) in Iraqi Kurdistan.

SWEDISH ADOPTION

Since the 1960s approximately 40,000 foreign-born children have been adopted in Sweden. Three of those children are mine. While most of the children have come from Korea, India, and Colombia, my daughter came from Iran and my two sons came from Thailand. Sweden has the largest population of intercountry adoptees in Europe and per capita (1 to 1.5 percent of the total population born after 1965) in the whole world (Hoksbergen, 1990). I adopted as a single woman, which is unusual; only 3 percent of the adoptions in Sweden are by single people, although there is no legal restriction against such adoptions.

Since I am a physician, I belong to the large group of adoptive parents who work in the health professions (17 percent of the mothers and 14 percent of the fathers in one of our Swedish adoption studies). Half the mothers and 20 percent of the fathers worked as teachers or in the health care professions, according to another study. In Sweden most adoptive parents are white-collar workers, 68 percent, compared to 45 percent in the total population, according to Swedish statistics for adoptees 1970-1979. As with most adoptive parents, I was older than the average biological parent when I got my children at thirty-five, thirty-seven, and forty years old. Forty-seven percent of adoptive parents were thirty-two years old or older when they adopted, according to statistics (Hjern, Lindblad, and Vinnerljung, 2002). My children were very young at arrival; the oldest was four months old. About half of the children who came to Sweden for adoption at that time were six months old or younger when they arrived (in 1969, 1971, and 1974; Cederblad et al., 1999).

WHY DID I ADOPT A CHILD?

The most important reason for my adoptions was that I did not have any biological children. I was divorced and had not managed to find a new man who was willing to create a family with me. I did not want to live the rest of my life without children. I was getting older, and the age limit for adoption in Sweden at that time was around thirty-five years old (for the first child—one could adopt a sibling at an older age since the authorities considered it beneficial for a child to have siblings). Because of this, I had to make a quick decision.

One thing that made the choice easier was that my sister had adopted a baby girl from Finland in 1967. I fell in love with that little girl! It was easy to fantasize that she could in fact have been my child—had I adopted her instead of my sister doing so. For me it was not important to have a Caucasian child. I had met children in Sudan in my professional work, and I knew color or race were not important to me. I very much agreed with the slogan of the only adoption agency in Sweden at that time: "Children need parents, parents need children." I felt strongly—and still do—that we are all a human family, regardless of birthplace. All children have the same need for love and tender care and the same capacity to grow and develop if they get it. They also have the same capacity to give love back to their caretakers, whether they are biological, adoptive, or foster parents. Of course, growing up in different countries can make it more difficult to have the same spontaneous mutual contact later in adult life than you can have with a small child, due to different religions and cultures, but with a small child the contact is so basically human that race, culture, and social background do not matter at all, in my opinion.

In our family we have a tradition of nontraditional parenthood. My maternal great-grandmother had many foster children and also used the income from the government for this to help support her sick husband and her biological children. My paternal great-grandfather was an orphan found on the doorsteps of a poor farmer's house. My paternal aunt's sister adopted an orphan girl from Chile who had been brought to Sweden by missionaries, who died soon after they came back with her. Also, as I mentioned earlier, my sister and her husband adopted a girl from Finland. The year before my first adoption they also adopted a boy from Yugoslavia.

I had many friends and colleagues who had adopted. In fact, I got the name and address of a person who could find an adoptive child at an orphanage in Tehran, Iran, from a psychologist at one of my former work sites who had herself gotten two children from Iran. It was thus by chance that my daughter Liv came from Iran. I did not have any preferences regarding the country of origin or the sex of the child, but I strongly wanted to adopt as young a child as possible. Through my child psychiatric training I had great respect for the research on attachment, and I wanted to have as good an opportunity as possible to develop an early, strong, mutual attachment to my child. Being a medical doctor I also knew that the lack of antenatal care, poor delivery conditions, risk of perinatal illnesses, and nutritional neglect could damage the baby's brain during a very vulnerable period in life. This was another reason why I wanted the child who arrived in Sweden to be as young as possible.

My second child came through the first private adoption agency in Sweden, Adoptionscentrum, which started in 1969. Before that there were only private adoptions, as with my daughter's, and adoptions of Korean children through the Swedish Board of Health and Social

Wellfare. That started during the Korean war, when Sweden ran a Children's Hospital in Seoul. My boy was the first child adopted from Thailand through that agency. Since he was the illegimate son of a young relative to the maid in the home of a Swedish woman who arranged adoptions for Adoptionscentrum, she informed me that I could adopt the child before he was born. I could choose a name to enter on the birth certificate. Because of that, he is the only one of my children who does not have a name given by the orphanage. I chose "Kim" because it is a common name in Asia, used by both men and women, and also because it is the name of a boy in one of the novels from India by Rudyard Kipling. He wrote about his boy-hero that he was "the small friend of the whole world," which I hoped that my Kim would be.

My third child also came from Thailand through Adoptionscentrum. This time the arrangements were more formalized. He was one of five children adopted at the same time from an orphanage. I went there together with the other parents and we all stayed at a hotel while the legal proceedings took place. This time I had asked to have a boy, since I thought it would be good for the two boys to support each other's masculinity, if they should grow up without a father.

EXPERIENCES EN ROUTE TO THE ADOPTION

In Sweden one has to have a permit from the social agencies in the municipality to adopt a child. A social worker makes a home visit and does one or two more interviews. One also needs a health examination by a physician. The social worker asks for permission to check that the adopting parent does not have any records of criminal charges or alcohol or drug abuse. She also contacts two reference persons chosen by the applicant, who can testify about suitability for becoming a parent and personal qualities in general.

Since that time the investigation of each applicant has been supplemented by a group meeting of future parents, held five times or more with the social worker so the parents can get more information about adoption and have a chance to discuss their decisions. Since practically all Swedish families who adopt do so because they cannot have biological children, it is considered crucial that they have worked through their disappointment about their infertility before adopting.

Exploring this issue is an important topic during the whole investigation.

The Swedish application, including the adoption permit, is then forwarded through the adoption agency to the social authorities or directly to the orphanage in the child's country of origin. Different countries have different legal routines. Muslim countries, such as Iran, do not have adoption laws. Because of that my daughter was adopted in Sweden according to Swedish law. Thailand, on the other hand, has an adoption law. Both my boys were therefore adopted in Thailand and the adoption was ratified in Sweden. All lost their citizenship when they were adopted, and I had to apply for their Swedish citizenship, which they got without having to wait for some years as other immigrants do.

COSTS OF INTERNATIONAL ADOPTION

In Sweden it is illegal to pay for an adoption. The only money that was paid for the private adoption was the airfare for the person who brought my daughter to Sweden. Adoptionscentrum took a small administration fee for their work, and I had to pay my own travel costs for my trips to and stays in Thailand. Voluntarily I also made a donation to the orphanage where my youngest son had lived for four months. I felt this was morally necessary as a contribution to all those children who remained there in very poor circumstances. The sum was not very large compared to their great needs, but many adoptive parents have done the same; added together these donations helped the staff to buy medicines and better-quality food, at least temporarily. Many adoptive parents have also formed support groups, which have helped the orphanages their children came from in a more permanent way by providing economic assistance annually for many years.

During the thirty years that have passed, intercountry adoption has become much more expensive. Adoptionscentrum and a few other private agencies, which have been authorized by the government to arrange international adoptions, charge much more now for their services. They have people employed to do the job; at the time when I adopted, it was done by volunteers. Their staff visit the adoption authorities and orphanages in the donor countries periodically and the foreign staff sometimes visit Sweden. Seminars are given regularly to professionals at the social agencies, who conduct the investigations. Meetings are arranged for adoption researchers. Information is provided for different professional groups, parents, and adoptees. What was, at the time when I adopted, spontaneous help between people who longed for children and staff at orphanages and hospitals who wanted orphans to get a chance to grow up in families of their own, has become both more corrupt and more professional. I witnessed that transition myself.

My daughter was brought to Sweden by idealistic people who wanted only to help children in need. My middle son was also adopted through a voluntary organization, but the legal process was handled by a Thai lawyer who later started to arrange adoptions in an unethical and illegal way, which made the Thai authorities cease international adoptions for a long time. When my youngest son was adopted, the procedure had already become more professional, which was good, even if it gradually made adoptions much more expensive. This is a dilemma. The many pitfalls in the area of international adoptions need professional handling, which will make them more expensive. Then families with lower incomes will hesitate, and adoption will become a way to create families for the upper middle class. In Sweden the government now gives an allowance that covers approximately 50 percent of the adoption costs. Adoptive parents have equal rights to paid "maternity leave" as biological parents do. If the child is older at arrival, one adoptive parent can still have one full year paid leave (which can be divided between the parents, as with biological parents). Neither of these benefits existed when I adopted. They developed gradually as the number of adoptive families grew and became politically stronger as an advocacy group. Other reasons were that the costs increased dramatically and that research confirmed that children who are older at arrival generally show more adjustment problems.

MY DAUGHTER—
DELIVERED AT STOCKHOLM AIRPORT

The arrival of my daughter was quite dramatic. I was contacted by the Scandinavian airline company and asked to pay the airfare for a person accompanying a child who would arrive only two days later. I was waiting for a message about the adoption for some time but had not heard from the woman for months. When I went to the airport, I did not know if I would be getting a boy or a girl, nor the age of the child! There were three adults arriving from Tehran with five children who were to be delivered to their adoptive parents at the airport.

My child was a baby girl who had weighed only one and a half kilos (3.3 pounds) at birth. When she arrived she weighed two and a half kilos (5.5 pounds), and she was developmentally similar to a newborn child. The Iranian pediatrician, who had taken care of her at a hospital in a poor section of Tehran, thought that she was well enough to cope with the long air flight. The decision was made hastily so she was ready to join the transport of the other children who had already been arranged. He thought that she had a better chance to survive and develop in the home of a Swedish doctor than in an over- crowded pediatric ward in the understaffed hospital. Her name was Soghra, meaning "the small one." I added the name Liv—"life." That a child so premature survived in Tehran in 1969 must have been a miracle. Probably the only reason was that the pediatrician, who had received his specialization training in Stockholm, was especially in- terested in the care of premature babies. Liv's mother, a young un- married girl, had run away from the hospital after the delivery.

Liv has suffered from some developmental delays that may be due to this difficult start in life. She started to walk a little late and she had very delayed speech development. She uttered only a few single words before three years of age. Her pronunciation was also poor, so she received speech therapy for several years. Now her speech is quite good. She was a slow learner at school. She has dyslexia, which still makes it difficult for her to read and write. She also has difficulty memorizing things that she learns in a theoretical way. Practical, con- crete learning is easier. Her school problems caused poor self-esteem, and she would comfort herself by overeating. This made her over- weight, which decreased her self-esteem even more. I moved her to a Steiner school, which is a school using a special education program based on anthroposophic ideas. They stress artistic, practical, and spiritual development as much as intellectual training in the school curriculum. That did not help much, however, except that I think that her self-esteem would have suffered more in a regular school. When compulsory school finished, when she was sixteen years old, we were both relieved. After that she studied at a cooking school for one year and had adult education with a special program for dyslexia for two years. She has been working for some years now in a school making school lunches. She likes her job and she is very much appreciated by her colleagues and the schoolchildren. She is still struggling with her weight problems but at present rather successfully.

Because of her learning problems and her overeating she was often depressed during her teens. She has always had many close girl-friends, but finding a nice boyfriend has been difficult. For many years she dated boys who had many problems themselves, such as alcohol or drug abuse, criminal behavior, and long-term unemployment. I have spent many nights worrying about where she was and with whom. Now at the age of thirty-two she has matured and has a steady relationship with a socially well-adjusted man without any psychiatric or antisocial problems.

MY OLDER SON—A HAPPY ENCOUNTER IN "THE LAND OF SMILES"

Kim was only two weeks old when we met at the small private nursing home where he was placed by the representative of Adoptionscentrum immediately after delivery at a Bangkok hospital, until he could accompany me to Sweden. It was a pleasant house, run by a nurse and quite well kept. He stayed there while the legal procedures were finalized. Everything went smoothly; the lawyer, who later became a crook, was still straight and very efficient. The only problem was to make Kim open his eyes when the passport photo was taken. The bright light made him close them and the photo had to show open eyes to be valid.

Our problems started when I brought him to the air-conditioned hotel room, where I stayed some days before our departure. He got a cold and started to have diarrhea, which got worse during the seventeen-hour-long flight back to Stockholm. When we arrived he was dehydrated. We had to go directly from the airport to a hospital, where he was admitted and given intravenous fluids. When he was discharged, he was prescribed mother's milk. I could collect a bottle of that every day at my local store, where it was delivered from the hospital. He is therefore one of very few adopted children who got mother's milk for four months after the adoption! He was a big boy when he was born, three kilos (6.6 pounds), and after his severe diarrhea episode he thrived on his mother's milk diet. In fact, he has always had excellent health, both somatically and mentally.

When Kim and I returned home, Liv was furious. She was extremely jealous for a long time. She was two years old and did not yet have the language to express her feelings, but her nonverbal language was very clear: "Get rid of that intruder!" She often tried to hit or pinch him, especially when I was feeding him. She cried and sulked a lot and demanded constant attention. In that situation it would have been much easier to be two parents! Kim was an easy child. He has always been calm and has adjusted easily to new situations and new people. He is very sociable and has always been a buddy among buddies. I was not surprised that he was chosen "soldier of the year" of his regiment when he served his one-year compulsory military duty in the Swedish army. Officers and his fellow soldiers selected him because he was ambitious in his duty and a dependable and cooperative member of the platoon.

Kim never had any problems at school scholastically or relationship-wise, but his interests were sports and crafts rather than theoretical subjects. He went to vocational school and trained to become an electrician. He has worked at that now for more than ten years. He met his future wife in 1994, at the age of twenty-two years. They moved in together after only a couple of months and have been living together since then. They have two lovely boys, four and a half and two years old, and a third child is due to be born soon.

Emmy Werner (Werner and Smith, 1992) defined "positive mental health" as being able to "work well, love well, play well and expect well" in the Kauai study. In my opinion Kim fits that definition. He is satisfied with his work and has a wonderful family whom he loves. He plays football and land hockey with a group of good friends whom he has known since his school days, and he is an optimist who seldom complains but looks forward to the future with confidence. Once when I was professionally very absorbed in a research project on the development of ethnic identity of internationally adopted teenagers, I asked Kim, "How do you feel? Do you feel Swedish or do you feel Thai?" He answered, "I feel ordinary."

MY YOUNGEST SON—
A LESS DRAMATIC START

Somkid—"the pretty one"—was four months old and lived in a large orphanage run by Catholic Thai nuns in a remote city in eastern Thailand. The institution was overcrowded and very dirty. He had severe scabies, which I treated immediately in Bangkok after consulting a Thai doctor. He prescribed much stronger doses than were recommended for infants on the instruction paper in the package of salve. As I did not want to poison him, I followed those instructions instead of the doctor's advice—which turned out to be a mistake, I realized, when the rest of the family started to itch after being home a couple of days. He seemed cured when we arrived in Sweden. (This time I had turned off the air-conditioning in my hotel room!) On arrival we went through the general health examination that is recommended for foreign adoptive children. It was then discovered that he also had salmonella. Because of that, my other two children were not allowed to attend their day care center temporarily and we all had to have stool examinations. While we were all at home washing our hands with special detergents and placing his diapers in a special container to be destroyed by the health authorities, we all started to itch. All of us now had got the scabies! The ointment used for treatment is very strong. It burns, especially when you get it in your eyes, which small children easily do. There was a lot of crying and a lot of washing, since all sheets and towels had to be washed each time we repeated the cure, and it had to be repeated quite a few times until we finally got rid of the scabies.

Apart from this nuisance, adding Somkid, to whom I gave the Swedish name "Love," to the family was easy. Liv made him her baby and pushed him in her doll pram. Kim accepted him in his typical way of easily adapting to new situations. Love is a more sensitive and self-reflective person than Kim, but he is also more aggressive. Both have experienced teasing for their foreign looks by other children. Whereas Kim ignored such situations or withdrew, Love fought. He has always been sensitive about being short at five feet two inches. (This was also the most common complaint of adopted teenagers when asked their opinions on their looks in a study that I conducted some years ago; Irhammar and Cederblad, 2000.) Since Swedes are tall, being short is often a problem, especially for boys. "Living in a land of giants" is how one Korean boy expressed his feelings. Love has been preoccupied with building a strong body as a compensation for his short stature. He has tried all sorts of martial arts. "It is my culture, Mom!" he argued, when I prohibited training in Thai boxing. He also started weight lifting and other fitness training early in his teens. He spent his compulsory military duty as a commando soldier—which was a voluntary choice. He served six months in Bosnia as a United Nations (UN) soldier, also voluntary. He has to prove to himself that he is a strong, masculine man.

Love chose to train to become a chef. He worked at different restaurants for some years, then suddenly decided to take a three-year course in hotel and restaurant management in Switzerland. To my great surprise he completed that. He was a very poor and uninterested student as a teenager. Now as a young adult he has succeeded in studying on a university level using English as the language of instruction and learning German and French along with business administration, accounting, etc. This shows how important personal motivation is! At present he works as an accountant on an American luxury cruiser sailing between Florida and Hawaii.

WHO AM I?

All adopted children, whether externally different from their adoptive parents or not, will at some time during their childhood, most often several times, ask themselves and their parents who they are, what their biological parents were like, why they were abandoned, and why they were chosen for adoption by these particular parents. How did my children handle these questions? Differently! Since my children belong to different ethnic groups, there was never an option/temptation to try to conceal that they were adopted and not my biological children. The question in "invisible adoptions," with parents and children belonging to the same ethnic group, of when to tell children that they are adopted never existed. My children knew from the beginning that they were adopted. (Strangely enough, in one of my studies on adoption, I met one Swedish family who claimed that their Korean child had never understood that she was not their biological child—and they wanted her to continue to believe so!)

When my daughter was about five years old she came home and asked me, "Did you buy me?" A playmate had told her that. I could honestly tell her "No," but, of course, with the rising adoption costs, it is today more unclear whether a child is in fact bought. The most difficult question to answer is, of course, "Why did my parents abandon me?" As do most parents of internationally adopted children, I explained that their parents were poor. I told them that the girls who were the mothers of Liv and Kim were young and unmarried, living in countries where a woman in that situation does not have the economic support from the municipality that a similar girl would have in Sweden. Their families could not help them either, due to special circumstances. In Iran the reason was—and still is—that an illegitimate pregnancy brings shame to the whole family. In Thailand, which is a bit more broad-minded, Kim's birth mother was herself an orphan whose parents were dead. Love was the sixth child of a poor farmer who could not even support the five children he already had. He left the smallest child in the orphanage as a way of saving him from starvation. These are complicated questions that need to be discussed many times during the childhood years on different levels according to the age of the child.

Liv sometimes cried during the Iran-Iraq war when the TV news reported about the many civilians who were killed, and she would say, "I think my mother has been killed now." How could I answer? Certainly not that her mother had probably died much earlier, because a young woman abandoned by her family in Iran does not have much choice other than to become a prostitute and most likely die quite young. Kim never asked about his mother. I am glad that he did not because there are some dark secrets about her that I know but would not like to reveal to him. Love has always been the one most interested in his biological and ethnic background. When he was a teenager he told me, "When I have grown up and got a job, I want to find my biological mother. I will send her some money, because you can support yourself, but she needs help."

GOING BACK: SEARCHING FOR ROOTS

Love is also the only one of my children who expressed a wish to return to his country of origin to try to trace his roots. I told him that I would help him to do that when he had finished his vocational training, because I thought that he should be a bit older since it would probably be an upsetting experience. I got a chance to arrange a suitable way for this to occur when I met a Thai social worker from Chiang Mai, a large city in northern Thailand. When she visited Adoptionscentrum in Stockholm in 1992, I told her that Love wanted to work, that he was a cook, and that he would like to stay with a Thai family for at least six months. She was interested in helping, as she worked with intercountry adoptions and shared my view that it would be a valuable experience for an internationally adopted child to return for some time to his or her country of birth. Some weeks later she wrote and told us that she had arranged a job at a first-class hotel-restaurant and that Love was welcome to stay with her family, which consisted of her, her husband, who was an agronomist, and their son, who was the same age as Love. I arranged to spend a six-month sabbatical at the Department of Psychiatry at the University of Chiang Mai, where I also could stay in a guest house for foreign researchers. I wanted to be available but not to interfere with his project. Love studied Thai part-time at a language school in Lund for six months before we left. This was on his own initiative. He also decided to use his Thai name, Somkid, while he was in Chiang Mai.

The experience was very successful. The family was middle class and had a rather Westernized lifestyle. They spoke English when Somkid's Thai was not sufficient. The culture clash was not too extreme. At the hotel-restaurant the Thai staff spoke only Thai, but the chef was French and the manager was Dutch. They used Somkid mainly in the European kitchen, since that was where they could profit from his Swedish training. He also had a chance to learn Thai cooking, which has proven valuable for his later work in Sweden. During the first weeks he came to me at the hospital every day for "debriefing," but as things got more familiar our contacts became more casual, such as visiting interesting sites together and other tourist outings, such as elephant riding and rafting.

Somkid realized from this experience that he was Swedish on the inside, even if it was a special feeling to walk on the streets and look like the rest of the people. He fell in love with a Thai girl at his job and fantasized about moving back to Thailand. The French and Dutch managers at his job encouraged him to go back to Europe and work for some years and then come back to a top position in Thailand, as they had done. In fact, Love worked during one of his trainee periods at the Swiss management school, in the year 2000, at a hotel belonging to the same chain of hotels in Pataya in southern Thailand. By that time he felt that it was too difficult to look like a Thai but not speak the language well or be culturally competent. He felt that the situation was too confusing, both for him and for his co-workers and the Thai guests.

During our stay in 1993 we also traveled to the orphanage from which I adopted him. It was not an orphanage anymore, but a school, still run by Thai nuns. They were very kind. They showed us around. I had brought Somkid's birth certificate, where the names of his biological parents and the name of his birth village were written. My plan was to take a bus to the village but not to try to find the family, since this could be a bit too sensitive. The parents might have told their relatives and neighbors that the child had died, not that they had given him away. The prioress said that we would never be able to find the village on our own. She offered to lend us the school car, their driver, and one nun who worked as an English teacher and could help us as an interpreter. Overwhelmed by their generosity, we happily accepted. The nun also thought it was OK to try to find the family.

After a long journey on narrow dirt roads across the rice paddies where there were no road signs, even in Thai, we arrived at a small village. The nun started to ask the inhabitants about the names of Somkid's parents. We were shown to the small Buddhist temple in the middle of the village. After some discussion and looking at the birth certificate, it became clear that the temple priest was a younger brother to Somkid's grandmother. He told us that both Somkid's parents were dead and that all his older siblings had moved to Bangkok or other cities to try to find work. A maternal uncle and his two children, Somkid's cousins, still lived at the village. They were working in the rice fields but eventually came home to meet us. After some time, all the villagers assembled in the temple. I had brought a photo album, showing Somkid's childhood in Sweden, as a gift. It was passed around and everybody was very interested. Then his relative, the priest, performed a Buddhist ceremony that is done to "welcome the spirit home." My son was given some rice and eggs to eat, and small, blessed, white threads of cotton were bound around his wrists

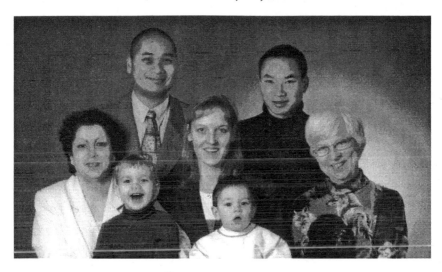

Marianne Cederblad with Her Children and Grandchildren

by everybody present. There was singing and praying and incense was burned. Somkid was deeply moved, as were I and his Thai relatives, who were sitting around him in the front of the temple. He wore those threads for a long time, and he still keeps them in honor of a very precious memory. After the ceremony we visited his uncle's house, where his parents had also lived and where he was born.

When Love later saw the photo that I took of him together with all the family members, he commented, "Now I can see that my short stature is genetic." He was nearly a head taller than anybody else in the family. It would have been possible to keep in contact with the family through letters, but Love never did. He did not visit the family during the two trips that he has made to Thailand since then. Maybe the encounter was too overwhelming or the answers to the questions about his background that he got were enough. The decisions are his.

Kim was not interested in trying to trace his biological family. He visited us in Chiang Mai for two weeks. He found it interesting but claimed that he was a Swede making a tourist trip, not a Thai returning to get in contact with his roots. At that time his relationship with his future wife was rather new. He was more interested in finding a beautiful ring for her than in getting in touch with his past.

REFLECTIONS

It is obvious from my description of the events around the arrival of my children that international adoptions are not projects for people who want to live their lives in a well-planned and smooth way but rather for the foolhardy. The adoption process has become a bit more bureaucratic and organized now than it was at the start of this enterprise. Luckily, at least in Sweden, adoptive families have been resourceful. Many have also been experienced travelers.

An omnipresent question: Is it ethically acceptable to move children from their ethnic roots and transplant them to a country where they will always be reminded that they are different, even if they feel Swedish? A lot of research has shown that the initial adaptation problems subside very quickly and that within a year most children are firmly connected to their families (Irhammar and Cederblad, 2000). The overwhelming majority also fare well during childhood. During their teens adopted teenagers are more preoccupied with thoughts about their biological and ethnic identities, but studies in Sweden—contrary to some in Holland—did not find any increase in behavior problems compared to nonadopted controls using an epidemiological approach (Cederblad et al., 1999). On the other hand, double the number of adopted teenagers were treated in child psychiatric units and three times as many were admitted in residential care for antisocial behavior, including alcohol and drug abuse, than Swedish nonadopted teenagers of the same age (Irhammar and Cederblad, 2000).

A recent study (Hjern, Lindblad, and Vinnerljung, 2002) of 11,000 adopted young adults born in 1970-1979 showed that, according to official statistics, intercountry adoptees had three times as many suicide completions, suicide attempts, and hospital admissions for psychiatric disorders, five times as many hospital admissions for drug abuse, and twice as many for alcohol abuse than nonadopted young adults of the same ages. The conviction for crimes was also about double. All the comparisons were to other Swedish-born young people in the same age cohort, adjusted for major sociodemographic confounders. Since the total number of such disorders is small, this still shows that the great majority of the adoptees fare well as young adults. Nevertheless, the data also show that quite a few adoptees cannot compensate for a very difficult start in life. Maybe adoptive parents also have to remind themselves not to expect their adopted children to function quite as well cognitively and socially as they would expect from their biological children. A Dutch study showed that there were more disrupted adoptions when the adoptive parents were white-collar workers than when they were blue-collar workers. That may be because the parents put excessively high demands on the children regarding such matters as school performance.

It is important for adoptive parents also to remember that each child has a history before the adoption moment. Studies have shown that the higher the age at adoption, the higher the risk of adaptation problems. This risk very much depends, however, on the number of separations and destructive events, such as abuse and neglect, that the child has experienced during that time (Cederblad et al., 1999). To be flexible and to have realistic expectations are important characteristics for prospective adoptive parents.

I was lucky to get my children very early in their lives. They are reasonably well adjusted and happy, but they have met racially based teasing at times, they have felt deviant at times, and they have sometimes brooded about their special situation compared to their friends. On the other hand, they would surely have had extremely difficult lives had they not been adopted but instead had grown up in their orphanages. Considering the alternative, it is not difficult to answer "Yes" to the question I posed. I have never regretted adopting my children. They have made my life very rich.

REFERENCES

Cederblad, M., Höök, B., Irhammar, M., and Mercke, A. M. (1999). Mental health in international adoptees as teenagers and young adults: An epidemiological study. *Journal of Child Psychology and Psychiatry, 40*(8), 1239-1248.

Hjern, A., Lindblad, F., and Vinnerljung, B. (2002). Suicide, psychiatric illness and social maladjustment in intercountry adoptees in Sweden: A cohort study. *The Lancet, 360*(August 10), 443-448.

Hoksbergen, R. (1990). Intercountry adoption coming of age in the Netherlands: Basic issues, trends and developments. In H. Alstein and R. Simon (Eds.), *Intercountry adoption: A seven country perspective* (pp. 247-260). New York: Praeger.

Irhammar, M. and Cederblad, M. (2000). Outcome of intercountry adoption in Sweden. In Selman, P. (Ed.), *Intercountry adoption developments: Trends and perspectives* (pp. 143-163). London: British Agencies for Adoption and Fostering.

Werner, E. E. and Smith, R. S. (1992). *Overcoming the odds.* Ithaca: Cornell University Press.

Chapter 9

A Perfect Lottery

Jehoshua Kaufman

PREADOPTION CONSIDERATIONS

My wife and I thought we would be perfect parents. We are well educated—a psychologist and a social worker, respectively—and both licensed psychotherapists with much experience working in child psychiatry. We actually already had some real experience as parents of a son of mine from a previous marriage. He is a wonderful boy now fourteen years of age, who is mostly well behaved and intelligent. We did not expect parenthood to be much different with adopted children, but, as we say in Sweden, "those who live will learn." Eight years and two adopted children later, we definitely have learned a great deal.

Although we were young at heart, our chronological ages were not so young. At the time of our application for adoption, I was thirty-four and my wife was thirty-nine years of age. Still far from being old, we were not really seen as young in the eyes of the main organization for international adoptions in Sweden, called Adoptionscentrum (AC).

Actually, we did not fit at all. Not only did we mismatch agewise, but most countries want the women to be under the age of thirty-five. The age of the man does not seem to be of much importance, as long as he is a good provider. Then there was the problem of morality. I was divorced and so was my wife. I already had a child, and I was Jewish. Not every country accepts Jews as recipients of their children, although this is not openly stated. Also, our marriage was of short duration; we had been married for only a couple of years when we applied. It is common in Sweden to live together for a few years before getting married, if you ever actually do take that formal step. This is not accepted in the process of adoption and, realizing this, we rather quickly took the necessary legal steps and got married.

Even so, we were initially told that our marriage was too short for us to be considered suitable by AC. However, at that time, the waiting list was so long that our marriage would have gathered considerable years before it was our turn. Nonetheless, we had good educations, lived relatively comfortably in a small city, and held well-paid jobs. These were factors in our favor.

"Why do you want to adopt?" was a frequently asked question at that time. For our close friends and for us the answer was extremely simple. We could not have children of our own. Not that we did not try, and try, and try again. First it was enthusiastic lovemaking to conceive a child, then in combination with pharmacotherapy, and, finally, after one or more years, in vitro fertilization (IVF). This is very expensive, complicated, and psychologically painful, often with no result.

I always wanted a large family. Remaining childless was not an option. I did have a child, but one did not satisfy my aspirations of a suitable size family. My wife was at least as committed as I was about this. We had talked about adoption from the time in our relationship when children became a topic. She had been pregnant ten years earlier, ending in a miscarriage, but even then it had taken six months of trying. She had also worked as a social worker and in that position had evaluated couples in our situation.

So for us, perhaps different from other couples, adoption was a possibility from the beginning, although we had started out hoping we could become parents biologically. Initially, adoption was the second-best option—at least for my wife. I saw some fascination in adoption and the thought of different colors, backgrounds, possibilities. I cannot really say why now.

Realizing our ages, and that time was against us, we decided to try adoption at the same time that we looked for medical solutions. This, we knew, was not recommended, but we saw no other alternative. Waiting for all other medical options to be tried would take at least two years, plus a further two years to wait in line for our turn to adopt, thus decreasing our chances due to the age requirements for adoption. Therefore, we applied to several different international organizations for adoption, but due to the aforementioned reasons they were all very pessimistic. We were told:

- You might get an older, handicapped child. You do not mind, do you?
- I do not think we can help you. Your marriage is too short. Have you really thought this through?

Ten years later we understand their questions and doubts, but at that time we became upset, sad, and felt humiliated.

To be accepted as adoptive parents we had to be evaluated by a social worker who met with us several times. She asked many questions. Some of them we found quite appropriate, such as our reasons for adoption, our experiences with children, our feelings about not having a biological child, religion, our professions, income, and health. Other questions seemed quite odd. What did the queries about our own childhoods, our relationships with our relatives, their opinions about adoption, our marriage, and our sexual relationship have to do with our ability to adopt and raise children? Being good citizens we tried to present good and reasonable answers.

During such an investigation, there are "right" and "wrong" things to say. For example, it is "wrong" to say that you are sorry you could not have a biological child; it is "right" to say that you have left all bad feelings about childlessness behind you. This was no problem for us, since we both had knowledge about and experience with psychological evaluations of different kinds. Still, we can imagine that some people can feel very confused and, worse, insulted by this kind of "cross-examination."

After these meetings, the social worker wrote a report. To this, she added the recommendations written by our relatives and friends. All this had then to be confirmed by the social board in our town. We also had to prove that we did not have criminal records.

We eventually adopted two children from different countries. The adoptions were entirely different, so we will write two very different stories. Three years passed between the adoption of the first child and the second. The first story is an emotional one, full of problems and difficulties. The second one was entirely different. Both have turned out well, but more about that later.

Economics of International Adoption

What an uninteresting subject, especially since this is about children. That was what we thought because we did have sufficient money or, if needed, we could borrow it. For those who are not in this position, adoption might be impossible, at least an international adoption. Going through a large organization, an adoption from eastern Europe cost at least $7,500 at that time, which was 1993. This was a lot of money, but only half the cost compared with an adoption from India or South America. Although we adopted through private channels, our costs were comparable. The second adoption from Latvia, three years later, involved the largest organization in Sweden and the costs were just slightly higher.

THE ADOPTION
OF CAROLINA MARTHA LINNEA KAUFMAN

As mentioned earlier, it was difficult for us to use an official organization. We instead contacted friends who had adopted privately from an orphanage in Poland. They gave us names and addresses, and we started the process of a private adoption. The contact recommended was a psychologist who was working at, and dedicated to, the orphanage. She became not only our contact but also a friend who helped and comforted us through the desperately long periods of "nothing happening but waiting."

The authorities in Poland turned out to be even more demanding, concerning paperwork and bureaucracy, than those in Sweden. They requested certificates about citizenship, marriage, criminal records, living conditions, medical reports, medical tests for venereal diseases, and our psychiatric conditions, and a report from the Polish consul in Sweden. By then, our original reports were starting to get old, so updates were needed.

After an initial contact over the telephone, they agreed to let us come to Poland for a brief visit. Based on suggestions from our friends, we brought oranges, teddy bears, and other toys. The reason for our visit was to establish a more personal contact and to assess the orphanage—How were the living conditions for the children? Did they have food? How was the psychological climate?—and then, of course, to determine what they wanted from us—More paperwork? Payoffs as bribery? Or what?

The Orphanage

The orphanage turned out to be a large building, more like a hospital than a place for children, with high ceilings, long and empty corridors echoing from every step and every word, rows of beds, toys more for looking at than playing with, and no room for individuality, at least not that we could see during our first visit. The children were between the ages of two and six years; they crawled around us, trying to make contact, holding our hands, smiling, stretching their arms, asking to be picked up.

The orphanage was obviously understaffed, and the few workers who were walking around talked in harsh voices. It was impossible not to cry at this experience, but showing tears did not seem appropriate. That had to wait for later. We made contact with the staff and the psychologist. They seemed to like us, and most of the children seemed to be doing OK despite the harsh circumstances. We were told by another adoptive parent that the orphanage, during the year prior to our visit, had so little money that the children went hungry for days. This year was better, but there were definitely no luxuries.

Assembling and translating our paperwork, we sent it to the orphanage and other officials and waited impatiently. We called them time after time to find out what was happening and to urge them to hurry. Then, finally, a couple of months later they made contact and invited us to an official meeting with a representative from the relevant authority. We traveled to Poland again and met a middle-aged woman who (very politely) asked us questions. Behold! Before going back to Sweden, we were told we were accepted. It was quick and no bribes were required.

Now it was for real. The next visit was focused more on which child we would get. The psychologist had already made her choice: a boy, three years old. She was certain, and we did not mind. She let us meet with him, although that is not the common procedure, and he seemed nice. We played with him and followed him through the day. Then we went back to Sweden to wait. Being rather optimistic, we did not expect it to take a long time—but it did.

To understand what happened next, one has to consider the system in Poland, at least during the early 1990s. Foster care was uncommon in Poland at that time. It was not uncommon for parents to have their children living in an orphanage for certain periods of time and for different reasons. This could go on for years. Even if the parents or relatives never visited the children, they could not be put up for adoption unless both parents agreed. If the children were left outside the door and there were no traces of their parents, the authorities still had to advertise, search, and investigate to find them. This could go on for many years before adoption could become a possibility, so children can wait for many years before becoming eligible for adoption. This boy, aged three, was not, in spite of the staff's wishes, formally available for adoption, and there was no way to know when he would be. Realizing this, the psychologist suggested another child, a girl. We returned to Poland with new presents and new hopes.

First Meeting

Martha was her name. She was born three years before we met her, the second child to a teenage mother and an unknown father. She was left outside the orphanage at the age of four weeks. As a result of poor or no care, she was tiny. In spite of her small body, she was described to us as very active and stubborn, which probably made her unpopular with her caretakers at the orphanage, and, for unknown reasons, she was slow in developing language.

We were extremely nervous while waiting in a separate room. She came in looking scared but at the same time very curious. She moved nervously around the room. Quickly checking our bags, her small hands went searching for candies. Chocolates from Sweden disappeared immediately, as did most other things. We were shocked by her intensity, her movements, and her appearance. Our attempts to make contact with her in these few minutes seemed to fail. We even bent down to her level to make eye contact, but to no avail.

Suddenly she noticed us, and we scared her. She ran into a corner and screamed, and that was that. The rest of the day we followed her around in the large building. After a while, she did let us get closer and help her with her food, give her things, and watch her while she played. Finally, she walked beside us, not smiling, but at least looking.

To say that we were worried is an understatement. What was this about? What kind of a child was this? Normal? Retarded? Autistic? We understood, through professional experience and knowledge, that children raised at an orphanage of this kind often have developmental problems affecting them both cognitively and physically. We also knew that they *usually* turn out all right after a couple of years. This child was definitely different.

What Made Us Decide to Continue?

The first incident happened when leaving Martha after dinner. We watched her walk away down the long, echoing corridor, a tiny child with a teddy bear in her hand. It was like seeing her walk alone into endless hopelessness, a terrible sight. Then, she looked back and, perhaps, smiled at us.

The second incident also followed dinner. All the children had to take a nap, so we took a stroll. Upon returning, we found Martha in an intense "discussion" with the staff about some shoes. She was crying and screaming—more out of anger than despair. We were told that she was very stubborn. Not being a favorite meant not getting any attention, no extra food, or other favors, but she was fighting, struggling to get her part of the world and not giving up. Both my wife and I found this inspiring. This was no "learned helplessness" or "depression." This was a struggling child.

The third incident occurred at the end of the day. We had a discussion with the psychologist about our thoughts, and she told us that during the day she had noticed Martha's position in the group change from lowest to a much higher position. In the eyes of the other children, she was on her way to becoming someone—someone with parents. We realized then that we could not say no; she was already a part of our family.

Before focusing on the process after she left the orphanage and up to the present, I would like to comment about pain. I am especially interested in this subject because it is a large part of my professional work. I work with chronic pain patients and have been doing this for some time, which may explain the reason for my interest in this incident. During one of our visits to the orphanage, Martha was playing with a group of children. They were running up and down a small slope and enjoying themselves. Suddenly, we saw her fall, and although she did not cry, we could see that she was hurt, as there was blood on her forehead. Before we could get to her, she stood up and started to run and laugh with the other children again. For us, with our experience with my son who screamed in pain over every little thing that might be hurting him, this was different. Was she not able to feel pain? Discussing this later we concluded that this must be a result of lack of attention. Crying is a behavior of communication, and if the result is no response, you stop crying and try to find other ways to communicate your experience. If you do not find any ways, you will stop trying. When we talked about these ideas with our friend the psychologist, she agreed. The children in general and Martha specifically were not spoiled with attention. Our hypothesis was confirmed very soon when Martha, realizing that it would lead to attention and comfort from us, started to cry and scream when hurt.

Who Was Martha?

So who was this Martha whom we adopted at the age of three years? We have already covered most of our knowledge about her background. Next, we left Poland with our daughter, hoping to live happily ever after! If happiness is being parents, we accomplished this goal, but everyone with children knows that giving birth is one of the easier parts. In that sense adoption is no different.

Physically Martha has been, and is, extremely healthy. Apart from a cold now and then she is hardly ever sick. Psychologically, though, it has not been so easy.

The Difficult Aspects

Martha, or Carolina, as we decided to name her, as she had both names, quickly became attached to us. We stayed in Poland for a week to complete all the legal arrangements but also to learn to know Carolina in her "normal" context. During this week she lived with us in a guest house around the corner from the orphanage. After two days, we started to get more than passing contact, and by our return home, it felt as if she was somewhat connected with us.

Similar to many other children raised in an orphanage, she eagerly approached most adults she could reach, but this was a behavior we were prepared for and could handle. Her activity level was extreme. Her hands and feet were all over everything. She ran all over the place. Sleeping was initially a problem. She could not be still long enough to fall asleep. Finally we found out that she could fall asleep lying on our stomachs. She had started to use the toilet before coming to us but that immediately stopped, and we had to use diapers.

Most child experts would say that these behaviors are more or less common for the first year or so, especially considering the age of the child when she was adopted and her background. Most of this we knew, but only theoretically. The reality was definitely not expected. Tired after the journey and the process of bringing her home, we found ourselves drained of strength. We had a child with the moving ability, curiosity, and strength of a three-year-old, but who was cognitively and socially only one year old. It was difficult, and after the first confusing weeks, we decided that she was developmentally only about a year and a half. We had to lower our expectations and work with one task at a time.

Writing this, I suddenly fear that perhaps my memory fails me. My wife agrees. I seem to have forgotten a lot of things. It did not take a couple of weeks before she became attached to us; it took more than six months. Yes, she did fall asleep on our stomachs, but not voluntarily. In our desperation to establish a relationship with her we used "holding" as a method, and she did not seem to like it—not the first time, nor the second or third! Weeks later, however, we could see that it did make a difference. She did not cling to our hands walking in town or at the beach, but we had to hold her hard, carry her, and keep her attention in different ways. It took a lot of ice cream cones, candies, and talks, but finally we made some progress. Perhaps this "failure of memory" is a salutogenic ability the human mind uses to help us survive difficulties. Concerning having and raising children, it certainly makes it possible for couples to have more than one child.

Years went by, and our family grew closer. Carolina had difficulty talking and concentrating; she struggled to find words and pronounce them. The speech therapist we consulted told us that these were normal problems, considering her background, and that we were over-concerned parents. We refused to accept this, and with support from the staff at her kindergarten, she got extra help from another speech therapist. Her speech improved, but her problems with concentration and extreme activity continued. She also got extra help for this at the kindergarten and even more at the preschool. Slowly we started to realize that she had learning problems that would probably not go away over time, at least not by themselves.

Together with the psychologist and teaching staff, we started to plan her first year in school. In Sweden children begin school at the age of seven years. It was decided that she would start in a smaller group with five pupils and two teachers. We felt very good about this and so did Carolina, who really looked forward to becoming a schoolgirl. It seemed to work out all right. She loved going to school, found friends, and liked different kinds of activities.

I do not want to idealize this period. There were many problems and worries, but they felt like "normal" problems. We met other people with biological children who were experiencing the same kind of difficulties. During this first year a cognitive and neurological evaluation was done. It turned out that Carolina had severe cognitive problems and that she would probably need special education. It was also suggested that we try some medication for her problems with attention and concentration. We agreed to this, and it worked out well. From one moment to the next she seemed to "clear" up and to look around with "new" eyes, and her ability to keep up with schoolwork increased enormously.

The Wonderful Aspects

So what were the beautiful moments that helped us over the hard times? It was nice to have another child in the family. Having her fall asleep on our stomachs and in our bed felt good to us. She tried to learn, and she tried very hard, repeating words, trying to accommodate to her surroundings. She did well with other children of her age or younger. A good part of this story is her relationship with her brother, Eli. Three years older, he was a proud big brother, looking out for his sister. He was trying to understand what was going on and to help out. Since we were not able to spend equal amounts of time and energy on him, he quickly decided to behave more maturely, at least sometimes. He tried to play with her and show her things, and she tried to accommodate. Then she started to tease him. Very surprising to us and to Eli, she fast became well acquainted with all his weak points and how to use them, too. These were more or less sibling quarrels, and dealing with them made us feel like all other parents with two or more children.

Carolina actually did well with other children. She found her place in groups, both at the nursery and in the neighborhood. She found friends to play with rather easily. Being a very active child, she preferred playing with boys, but that did not worry us. Seeing all of this made us hopeful. It enabled us to look beyond the daily struggles to see her progress. She got rid of the diapers and spoke her first words. From the outside these might have seemed small steps, but for us they were miracles. Getting back to work, enrolling Carolina in day care, parents' meetings, and obtaining extra help for her in preschool—all of these things helped us to feel like we were one of many families.

Most fascinating is that her stubbornness in combination with her strong will and desire to learn and to be like everyone else are still within her. Even though she screamed and cried about homework and we found it terrible to do it with her, she was always eager to try and never gave up. If we gave up because of her crying, she would immediately say, "No! Let's try a little bit more." Even if she is not able to follow the normal curriculum, she can function well in a special education group, where she is one of the best. So school did work out well and, perhaps, that is what made us apply for another child. This time we intended to go the "normal" way. Times were different. Recession had made adoption an expensive activity. The queues were smaller. Our marriage was of a longer duration, and potential countries with children available for adoption were more plentiful. Also, our energy level was not as high.

JONATHAN EDGAR ERIK JOINS THE FAMILY

This time, in 1994, the discussion with AC went entirely differently. They were polite, interested, and very positive. They could see no problems in helping us with this adoption. Still, it took nearly two years from our first application to the authorities until Jonathan came home with us.

From the start we were very open concerning the country of origin of our next child. Although it was now possible to have a child from India, different aspects of our own situation made Russia and Eastern Europe seem the best choices. The number of orphans in the former Soviet empire was enormous, their orphanages were full, and there was a need for parents.

This time was entirely different for us, on a personal level as well. We were as committed as before but much more patient. Our days were full of activities, we already had children who needed our attention, and we had learned a lot from the first adoption. We decided to apply through several different organizations. This way we would hopefully have some degree of choice. The expense would grow since all organizations demanded a large fee just to apply, and, over time, as the applications were worked through and translations done, the cost would increase even more, but we decided that it was worth it.

After a year, we started to receive suggestions about children ranging in age from three to five years. Unfortunately, their medical situations worried us to the degree that we decided to pass. We consulted friends who were physicians, and they all advised against adopting children with severe medical problems, even if the adoption organization described the problems as curable. We did not dare to risk any more worries. As we saw it, even if the child seemed to be in good physical and emotional health, there might be problems later due to the child's background, and we wanted to start out as good as possible. This may sound logical and clear, but it took a lot of thought, many discussions, and more emotional pain to say no. Questions such as "What right do we have to say no to a child?" and "How do we know that the next possible child, if there is one, will be better?" faced us. It was not easy, and we hope that we will not face the same kind of dilemma in the future.

AC regularly publishes a newsletter with pictures of happy families, articles about different projects in the third world, and information on adoption. It also includes a page with photos and descriptions of children for whom it is difficult to find parents or who need parents very quickly. I usually went through this page thoroughly but always decided that none were for us. Then one day I (or was it my wife?) saw him. A cute baby boy, one year old, with sparkling eyes and a wonderful smile. Reading the text, we found out that he had a problem with his heart. The disease was described as easily treated in Sweden, but a fatal problem in Latvia. Suspicious after our earlier experiences, we called the AC, got a better medical description, and talked with a lady who had actually met him. She was happy to hear that we were interested but told us that a couple had already called up and were therefore first in line.

Our medical specialists agreed that the described problem was no big deal for a Swedish heart surgeon, but that there might be an urgent need for an operation. We called the AC again and expressed our willingness to adopt this child if the other couple relinquished their position. A few days later we were eagerly waiting, although we did not talk about it to avoid any unnecessary disappointment, when the telephone rang and we were parents again.

Until that moment we were not sure about our decision. Could we handle another child with problems? But as soon as we knew this child was ours, his health status was important only in the sense that it had to be dealt with as quickly and as safely as possible.

Our previous experience with adoption was that everything took an extremely long time, but this time was different. Everyone seemed to be eager to get all the paperwork done. The formal decisions were made quickly, and the travel arrangements were put in order. The reason was, of course, concern over Jonathan's health. As parents, we tried to find out as much medical information as possible. We talked to doctors, arranged treatments, and prepared for some hospital visits and surgery. We found out that nothing could be confirmed before the child had arrived. A son of our friends was born with heart problems, and we had long discussions with them about such conditions. This turned out to be one of the most valuable relationships of this period. They eased our minds about issues concerning hospitals, doctors, and surgery.

Another Type of Orphanage

A few months later we were on our way to Riga in Latvia; it was springtime 1996. The service was excellent: someone picked us up at the airport, drove us to the hotel, and presented us with a program for the next three days, ending with us going to the airport for our return to Sweden with Jonathan. On this tour Carolina was with us. She was very excited about getting a baby brother and traveling abroad to pick him up. Eli, our older son, was excited too, but he could not come with us. Carolina talked continuously about the new sibling and prepared herself and us for the newcomer. She bought toys for him, helped furnish his room, and did all kinds of things to show her excitement.

Understandably, we were all eager to meet him. The orphanage was just outside Riga. It was a nice, one-story building surrounded with trees and grass. The atmosphere seemed relaxed, and the staff we met were nice and smiling. It was very different from our Polish experience. There were no other children at our visit, which lasted for about three hours and ended with us leaving with this smiling and curious child in our arms. During these few hours we got to meet him, comfort him, feed him, and dress him. Initially he avoided us and screamed, but Carolina picked him up and somehow he calmed down. After that, he became very curious and active in our interaction.

This was very different from what we had expected—not only the surroundings and the interpersonal context, but also the child himself. We had expected, due to his heart problem, a tired and weak boy, but Jonathan seemed to be just the opposite. He had a good appetite and tried to reach out for everything new. He did not seem tired at all. An example of his activity level was that, during this first twenty-four hours of our lives together, he did not fall asleep until the middle of the night. He tried every new food we gave him, taking it into his mouth but not swallowing, merely tasting and testing and spitting it out. He examined every geographical space he could find—our room, the corridors, the dining room, and other accessible spaces. Outside the hotel, he was much more cautious, merely looking around with wide eyes from his baby carriage. Much later, we understood that he probably had never been outside on his own. The first beautiful day of spring, perhaps a week after our homecoming, we went out in the garden. When we tried to put him down on the grass, he cried desperately and clung to us. A few hours later, after carefully examining the grass, he began to expand his outside world. Our guess is that because of his medical problems he was never allowed outside on the ground. After this first encounter with the outside world, he became an outdoor child, crawling on every outside surface—grass and mud gave him the same amount of pleasure.

Jonathan's Background

From what we could see, Jonathan had been treated well at the orphanage. The staff seemed attached to him, and we noticed a few tears as we left. He was well fed and open and trusting of other adults and children.

We know a little about his parents and their situation. Jonathan is one of at least four siblings in a very poor family. He came to the orphanage when he was only a few months old and apparently not very healthy. He has had numerous medical examinations and he behaves absolutely marvelously in a medical setting. When other children cry and yell, Jonathan just seems to accept the doctors, nurses, and whatever they do to him. We seem to be more upset than he.

Health, Health, and Health Again

We were very occupied with Jonathan's health. We had been told that his heart might have problems handling the trip to Sweden. During our first days together we were continuously aware of him. Does he breathe? Does he look tired? Is he too active? The doctor's appointment was just two days away, but it felt like a long time. He was thoroughly examined at the hospital and we waited in tense silence for the results. We were as surprised as the doctors seemed to be. There was a heart problem—a small hole between the two chambers—but the hole was smaller than described in the documents we had received and did not seem to affect him whatsoever. There was no need for surgery, at least not for the next few years, and the doctors were relatively optimistic about the future. Perhaps there would never be a need for an operation. To this day (Jonathan is now seven), there have been no problems relating to his heart.

Jonathan was a wonderful child, cuddly and usually in a good mood. Everyone loved him, and that is still so. He had no problems sleeping. He remained active and enjoyed being outside. He examined every new surrounding curiously. He did not always stay as close as we would like him to. He had a hard time being still at gatherings and at the lunch table, which created some problems in kindergarten.

Jonathan was also slow in developing language skills. A year after his arrival we found out that he had problems hearing. The doctor's theory was that untreated inflammations had caused this. A small operation was of big help for his hearing, and then his speech improved rapidly.

OUR THREE CHILDREN

Some researchers on family development state that having a member join or leave the family is one of the biggest stress factors in life. Looking at Eli, the oldest son, I realize that he has been through a lot of stressful changes in his life. More than others? I do not know. Certainly having two new siblings is a change, but then there is the question of how getting adopted siblings is different from having biological ones.

Looking at it from this present perspective, I cannot really see any differences. Preparation time is about the same or even longer. Eli even got to see a picture of his brother before they actually met. It was not babies whom we brought home, but small children, and they are of course different. Are the differences significant? We doubt it. I talked to him about it the other day. I asked if he would like to write a few pages about getting and having adopted siblings. He told me he did not mind, but he could not really see that his situation was any different from that of his friends with siblings.

For Carolina, to get a younger brother must have been very natural. She also participated in the "birth process" by going with us to Latvia. From the beginning they interacted as most siblings do. Carolina liked him very much, but after a while, when she found us overly occupied with him, she got jealous and once she suggested that we should take him back to where we got him. This is history; now they are like most siblings. They tease and play with each other. The smaller looks up to the bigger. The bigger one tries to teach the smaller and he tries to learn from her. When they are bored they fight, and when the fight is over they play again. Sometimes we feel that parenthood is overwhelming, but so do our friends now and then.

Both Carolina and Jonathan are blond and their features are not only Caucasian but also very similar to the rest of the family. I have family pictures with all the children on my desk at work. People tend to talk about how they all look like me. Their expression of surprise is honest when I, sometimes, explain that two of them are adopted. Sometimes I do not explain because I like the idea that they resemble my wife and me. Occasionally we speculate that if they were of another color, that would have reminded all of us about their background, creating a feeling that they are different. Talking to friends with adopted children from South America, I find that they usually do not think about their children or their family as being different from other families.

TELLING CHILDREN ABOUT THEIR BACKGROUND

With our professional experience, we are well aware that knowledge of one's background is a part of developing a sense of identity. We took pictures in Poland and in Latvia, and we made albums of the children's playmates, caretakers, and official papers. We talked with them about their countries of origin. We tried to create stories for them from our knowledge of their backgrounds and what happened to them before the adoptions, stories that would make life and adoption understandable.

Although Jonathan has shown little real interest, Carolina has been very interested, at least periodically. She asks questions about her mother and about herself as a baby. She is apparently trying to create a story of her own, filling in the gaps we have not been able to. She keeps asking us questions:

- Did I speak Polish when we met?
- Did you meet my mother?
- Can we go visiting?

A lot of these questions are difficult or impossible for us to answer. Sometimes the answer has a negative connotation because of our knowledge of the actual history, and that makes us hesitate. We find other related subjects in order not to be negative in talking about her background, but it is a difficult balancing act. Sometimes we ask ourselves if it is right to hide things from her. In time we will probably have to tell her everything we know.

We expect that both children will probably become more interested as they grow older. In our minds we are preparing a trip to both Poland and Latvia to visit the orphanages, towns of birth, and important places in the countries. Perhaps we can get together with people who knew the children or their relatives.

What have we done concerning our adopted children's relation to their respective countries of origin? We are still members of AC, the organization for international adoptions. This organization arranges meetings with other families, such as gatherings and excursions to the countryside, lectures, and other events that help families enjoy and deal with their situations. So far we have attended only a few of these. This summer there will be a gathering with families who have adopted children from Latvia and we hope to attend. Most adoptions from Poland were made privately and that usually means that there is no network of families or organizations to arrange gatherings. For Carolina we will have to find other ways of connecting her to Poland, if she wants that later in her life.

THE PRESENT

At present most things are going well. Jonathan is in first grade and Carolina is in fifth grade. They are in different schools because of the age difference. Carolina rides her bike to school while Jonathan goes with me every morning. Both of them enjoy learning, although Carolina still has considerable learning difficulties. She enjoys sports and plays most games involving a ball. Once a week she practices squash at a nearby club. She has a strong need for physical activities and enjoys them on her own or in groups. Jonathan has, at least so far, very little interest in sports but loves being out in nature. We often go to the forest for excursions, and he explores every creek, swamp, and meadow that we pass. Jonathan enjoys listening to facts about nature and seems to easily remember names of plants and animals. He joined the scout movement and he likes the ideas and enjoys the activities.

As we indicated, both children have had some problems in school, especially with concentrating and being still. Carolina has obvious learning difficulties. Luckily, the Swedish society is very good in meeting children's special educational needs. Carolina attends a special class with only eight children and three adults, while Jonathan gets extra attention from a teacher's assistant. Carolina will probably need this help most of her years in school. The educational system provides this assistance up to the tenth grade and then also in the gymnasium. That makes us feel very safe for the future. Jonathan's need for his assistant is decreasing, and at present she is needed only in the classroom situation. In smaller groups, during breaks, or in the more leisure-oriented parts of the afternoon, he does well on his own. This was not the case in the beginning of the school year.

So are these problems somewhat connected to adoption? We do not really know. As a psychologist I followed five or six adopted children during the early 1980s when I was working at a child guidance clinic. These children, who were all from different orphanages in Poland, had problems with concentration. Although these problems were of different levels of severity, all required special attention in the children's preschool and school years. I kept track of the children for a few years. At the same time I was in contact with a pediatrician in another area in Sweden. He had followed a group of fifteen children with the same background who had arrived in Sweden ten years earlier. I learned that the children he met had the same kinds of problems. After ten years, though, nearly all of them were doing much better. A lot of resources and efforts inside and outside of school were put into helping them handle their situation, and these efforts seemed to make a difference.

One can hypothesize about the reason for these problems. All of the children discussed were between one and a half and four years of age upon arrival in their new homes. They all came from orphanages and were described as passive and emotionally and cognitively under-developed. The orphanages were described as poor and with too few caretakers. It might be that a child under such circumstances does not develop adequately, but upon achieving a better situation, the child's development improves. I have a hypothesis that this development happens very quickly and that the attention deficit is more a result of this improvement. This idea has been a useful one for my wife and me. It has kept us hopeful and looking for good signs.

We do not see ourselves as special. Our identity is not "adoptive parents," and our children do not see themselves as special. When we meet other families with adoptive children we do talk with them and discuss background and experiences. We do not find our children doing this. Meeting other adopted children means nothing special to them, although this reaction might change later. For a while we tried to read children's books with adoption themes, but this was not well received by our children. We will simply wait for this theme to be raised by them one day.

THE ADOPTION PROCESS

Should Adoption Be Different?

During the process of adoption we often talked about our experiences. We used to tell each other, especially during bad moments, "When this is over, we will write a book about it!" Terrible periods lay behind us. Life is slowly blurring our bad feelings, and good experiences replace these feelings with gratitude. It was not the way it should have been, but it worked out all right. The past is the past, and the future will carry happy moments as well unhappy ones. That book about our terrible experiences will never be written.

Looking at the procedures for accetpance as adoptive parents, we sincerely think that these procedures should be changed. It is not appropriate to look for the perfect parents; good-enough parents are definitely enough. Thinking about the orphanage that our daughter came from, we hope that there soon will be prospective parents who are allowed to take all the children away from there. We listen to the radio news telling us that about 2 million children live without appropriate care in Russia, many of them on the streets. Newborn babies are killed because they are of the wrong gender or their mothers have a hopeless living situation. These children are in dire need of parents. Excluding addicts, pedophiles, and other undesirables, let all others, young and old, poor and wealthy, of all colors, alone or in different kinds of relationships, become parents if they want to. This will improve the situation for these children. Perhaps they will then receive some love and a platform for better lives.

In Sweden, discussion now centers around this issue. Should homosexual couples be accepted as adoptive parents? No data indicate that gay people are not good parents. The only reason I can see not to accept nontraditional adoptive parents is political. We think suitability should be evaluated by removing those who are unsuitable and accepting the rest.

Our Personal Adoption Process

Could we have done something differently in the process? Perhaps. Writing about this I think about the groups that were formed to prepare prospective adoptive parents. We never attended. We felt somehow that we were different, perhaps better qualified because of our professional status and experience, and having chosen another way to adopt. Looking back, I regret that we did not attend. It might have been beneficial to meet experienced adoptive parents. We would certainly recommend joining such a group to anyone who plans to adopt. It is not necessary but it might be helpful.

Would we recommend to others that they adopt? Yes, definitely. As mentioned, children need parents and parents need children, so it is a perfect match. It will not necessarily always be perfect, but life seldom is. There has been some research done on "what happened with our adopted children." Professor Marianne Cederblad (now retired) at the University of Lund did some interesting follow-up on this issue. The fear was that these adopted children would be more often in need of psychiatric help and more prone to develop social and psychiatric problems as adults. This was correct. Two percent out of the population of children raised in their biological families were in need of psychiatric help while 4 percent of adopted children had the same need—twice the amount. Still, 96 percent do all right. If a lottery offered a 96 percent probability of winning a nice prize, most of us would definitely go for it.

Chapter 10

Adopting from Eastern Europe 101

Karen Klein Berman

> Once upon a time there was a baby girl living in Russia who needed a mommy and a daddy . . .
>
> Once upon a time there were a mommy, a daddy, and a little son living in America who wanted a baby daughter and a baby sister . . .

Thus begins the story that I have repeated so many times to my daughter, now nine years old, who was adopted from Yoshkar-Ola, Russia, at the age of eighteen months. I am writing this chapter as the mother to two wonderful children and also as chair of the not-for-profit organization Families for Russian and Ukrainian Adoption (FRUA). My goal is to share the experience of my family's adoption journey, as well as to share some of what I have learned about the adoption process in my many years of being active in the adoption community.

Probably the most important bit of wisdom that I can offer is: *Do your research.* No one else can tell you everything you need to know, and no one else can tell you all the questions you will need to ask. Keeping that message in mind, I hope this chapter will add to your base of knowledge about the adoption process and, should you become an adoption professional or decide to adopt, help you toward a successful, life-changing adoption experience.

DECIDING TO ADOPT

It was December 1993. My husband, Jeff, age thirty-five, and I, age thirty-four, already had a biological son, Matthew, who was four years old at the time. We were living in Washington, DC; Jeff was an attorney at a large New York law firm, and I was a stay-at-home mom. I held a master's degree in education and previously had been a high school teacher and a group facilitator. After two years of infertility, the chances of us having a second biological child were becoming more and more remote. We always knew that we wanted to have two children, and we wanted a sibling for our son before he got much older. The strange routines of infertility treatments—such as sneaking into a restaurant ladies' room during dinner so Jeff could give me my daily injection of Perganol, and getting lots of knowing looks when we came out—made us question what we were doing. The hormones that I had been taking were making me quite moody and anxious and putting my health and relationships at risk. Jeff was the first to bring up the idea of adoption. He was tired of the medical intervention and the risks involved. We both knew that we would love to have a daughter, since we already had a son. That December we stopped the infertility treatments and began investigating the adoption alternative—full speed ahead!

To be unable to conceive a child when you want to is to lose control of an important part of your life. It leaves a feeling of helplessness. I discovered that one of the great advantages of choosing adoption over infertility treatments is knowing that you will have a child eventually. Control is regained and the helplessness disappears—and that is just the beginning.

Where to Adopt

We began to focus on where we would look for a child to adopt. The first decision was whether to adopt from the United States or internationally. We had three main reasons for quickly deciding to pursue an international adoption. First and foremost, we were aware of the desperate situation of institutionalized children in some countries and saw an opportunity to help address a real need. Second, because our son Matthew was already nearly school age, we wanted to act quickly, and we knew that trying to adopt an American child often involved being on a very long waiting list. Finally, it was very important to us, for our own emotional well-being as well as for Matthew's, to be able to turn the page and begin our new lives the moment we brought our adopted child home. Adoption laws in the United States do vary, but overall they tend to discourage adoption by favoring the rights of biological parents over the rights of adoptive parents, and many states' laws recognize a right of biological parents to revoke their earlier consent to an adoption. We knew ourselves well enough to know that the threat of losing our adopted child would be more than we could handle, and so adopting an American child was crossed off our list of possibilities.

The next step, then, was to decide in which country to focus our efforts. We considered China, Latin America, and Russia and ultimately chose Russia. Jeff's family and my family both have roots in Russia and Eastern Europe, so we both feel a connection to the Russian culture and people. We also decided against the additional complications involved with adopting a "minority" child. Among other things, we believed that we could do a better job raising our adopted child to be familiar with her own cultural heritage, and making that cultural heritage part of our everyday lives, if we adopted from Russia instead of from China or Latin America. In the end, when we considered the hundreds of thousands of orphaned children living in institutions throughout Eastern Europe, Russia's relatively "modern" approach to the rights of adoptive parents, and the period of less than one year during which most Russian adoptions are completed, Russia turned out to be an easy choice for us.

Selecting an Agency

Next we needed to find an adoption agency that was right for us. At the time we adopted in 1994, the choice of agencies was more limited than it is today. Now, with so many agencies offering international adoption services, the choice can seem overwhelming. Selecting an agency can be easier, however, if you keep in mind a few basic considerations and discuss them with the agency up front. Do you want to work with a large agency that may have more contacts and be able to refer a wider choice of children for adoption, but that has too many clients to offer much in the way of personalized service, or a smaller agency that cannot offer the same selection as a large agency but that has a more intimate, personal touch? Does the agency provide pictures, videos, and medical records of the children being placed for adoption? Will the agency support your decision to turn down a referral that does not meet your expectations and continue working on your behalf to find a comfortable match? Does the agency work in a number of countries and regions in case a particular area becomes closed to international adoptions as a result of unexpected political or diplomatic events? What are the ages of the children being referred by the agency?

Most important, talk to as many people as possible to get a variety of experiences and references. Make contacts through support groups, Internet chat rooms, and word of mouth. We found our adoption agency through a family member who had adopted four children successfully. It was a smaller agency, which I liked. There was always someone answering the phone, and they knew their orphanages and other Russian contacts—agency representatives, "facilitators," and orphanage directors—very well.

Now that we had settled on an agency, we began filling out forms, forms, and more forms—fingerprints, criminal record checks, autobiographies, multiple interviews with social workers, paperwork for immigration and naturalization, and notaries, notaries, and more notaries. All are part of the process, which becomes more or less a part-time job. For the required home study, we had a total of four interviews with a social worker: individual interviews for my husband and me, together as a couple, and finally at home with our son. The purpose of these interviews, of course, was to provide a professional opinion of our fitness as parents and our ability to provide a good home for an adopted child. This continues to be a critical element of all adoption procedures.

FINDING A CHILD

While all the paperwork is being done, the real search for a child begins. We told our agency that we were looking for a girl between the ages of one and two years old and wanted to be able to see photos, a video, and medical records before making a decision. We thought a young toddler would be right for us because our son was already four years old and we did not particularly want an infant. It would be nice for Matthew to have an instant playmate, and for us all to be able to sleep at night! We requested pictures and medical records because we were looking for a healthy child.

This brings me to a very important part of the adoption process, and the part where research is absolutely mandatory. Each family must decide what its own comfort level is when considering the health of the child. The health risks involved in adopting from Eastern Europe are well known, and the more you educate yourself, the higher the chance of a successful adoption. Poor prenatal care, alcoholism, poverty, and environmental contamination are prevalent in this part of the world and can contribute to health risks in children. Many health professionals now practice in the field of international adoption and can help you learn what to look for, what the potential risks are, and how you can minimize them. Medical/educational conferences take place throughout the year all over the country, and other resources are available as well, for example, support groups such as FRUA and Web sites with a wealth of information. I do not mean to scare anyone off but only to stress that to be well informed is to increase dramatically the chance of finding the right child for you.

After waiting three months, we received a phone call from our agency. I recall that it was a snowy February day. The agency had a video of two Russian girls, both thirteen months old, who were in need of a family. I begged my agency to send the video to my house right away, since waiting patiently is not one of my strong points. So, through what seemed to be at least a foot of snow, a driver made his way to my house with video in hand. It was the middle of the afternoon and I was at home by myself. I remember sitting on the floor of my bedroom watching the video of two little girls with tears running down my face. It was hard to believe that one of them would one day become our daughter, and we knew that whichever of these beautiful little girls we did not choose would be adopted by another loving family.

Seeing pictures of your child for the first time is an emotional event, but it also involves another important piece of homework. Take any videos, photos, and medical records that the agency provides and have them evaluated by a physician whose specialty is international adoption. There is a small but growing number of specialists throughout the country, but it is not necessary to live nearby because most of these physicians will do consultations over the phone if you send all of the pertinent information. Your local pediatrician typically will not have the knowledge or experience to do an evaluation from the limited information available, so I stress the importance of consulting a specialist who will know how to look for evidence of fetal alcohol syndrome/affect, cerebral palsy, developmental delays/disabilities, retardation, attachment disorder, and other medical issues found in the institutionalized child population.

After going through this process, we chose our daughter. We were very fortunate that the specialists we consulted believed that she was at low risk for any of the more serious potential medical issues. Although we informed our agency of our choice within a week of receiving the video, it is essential not to be rushed through the medical evaluation process and to work with an agency that allows time to make this very important decision.

Then we began waiting—waiting for the adoption and immigration paperwork to be completed, waiting for the Russian government to issue travel visas and give us the okay to travel to the orphanage and release our daughter to us, waiting for the U.S. government to issue entry visas—waiting, waiting, waiting. The adoption process teaches patience, or at least requires it. Once we chose the thirteen-month-old girl from the video to be our daughter, she began to grow in our hearts. We watched the video almost daily, and the waiting was not easy. She was our daughter and we wanted her in our home.

During this waiting period we needed to decide what to do about a name. The little girl had been given the name Angela in Russia, though we do not know by whom. We decided to use Angela as her middle name and to give her a new first name, realizing that she could always go back to Angela in the future if she so chooses. We had a few names in mind and decided to get our son's input. At the time a new character had been introduced on PBS's *Sesame Street*. This spunky, energetic, lively, orange-furred girl with pigtails was Zoe. Matthew decided that Zoe was his choice. To this day he is very proud that he was able to name his little sister, and she thinks it is pretty cool that she was named by her big brother! Deciding what to do about a name is a personal decision that each family needs to make. All children arrive with Russian given names, and it is up to the adoptive parents to decide what they would like on the birth certificate. We felt that her Russian name was part of her roots and heritage, so we wanted to keep it for her.

We began making travel preparations. After careful consideration, we decided that I would stay home with Matthew, and Jeff would travel to Russia to bring our daughter home. We were fortunate to have this choice—the local adoption procedures in our case did not require both adoptive parents to appear, but in many places in Russia it is not possible for only one parent to travel. I knew I would be sacrificing the experience of going to our daughter's orphanage and being part of her homecoming, but we felt it made more sense for me to stay at home with our young son and get everything ready for his new sister's arrival. For Jeff, this made possible a very special experience. He would go halfway around the world to pick up his little princess and bring her back to Matthew and me. It would be a wonderful bond that the two of them could, and will always, cherish.

We were told that Jeff would be able to travel by the middle of April, so we packed suitcases and Jeff made plans to take some time off from work. Jeff would be traveling with two other families adopting children at the same time, including the other little girl from the video, who would be going to her new home in California. Then April came and we were told that there would be a delay—one of the three children had become sick and they were all in quarantine. This was followed by another delay while local officials decided whether the three children, all better now, were too healthy to be adopted by foreigners. Complications and postponements have to be expected when dealing with international adoptions. Luckily, many airlines now offer special rates for adoption trips as well as flexible tickets that allow for date changes.

Finally, after the May 1 Russian holiday, we were given the go-ahead and Jeff was off to Russia with a suitcase full of toys for the children living at the orphanage, as well as gifts for the orphanage staff and local officials. Jeff brought along a camera and film to record his journey, plus warm clothes, a suit for court appearances and other official business, a stash of protein bars he hoped he would not need to eat, and a small pharmacy's worth of medicines, including antibiotics and vitamins, to leave behind at the orphanage. He also traveled with $10,000 in cash hidden under his clothing, strapped to his waist, to give to Dmitri, our Russian "facilitator." (Altogether, we spent nearly $25,000 on our daughter's adoption. The money went to pay the adoption agency's fees, travel expenses, home study expenses, and fees for processing visas and other documents. As for the $10,000, Dmitri didn't tell us where it all went, and we were just as happy not to know.)

While Jeff was traveling, Matthew and I prepared for the arrival of the new addition to our family. Matthew helped in getting Zoe's room ready and buying necessary baby equipment. We read books together about being a big brother and about adoption. When adding any sibling to a family, whether adopted or biological, there is an adjustment period for all family members. Matthew needed to get used to the idea that he was going to have to share Mommy and Daddy in exchange for having an instant playmate. At the age of five he was so ready to be a brother that there were not many problems.

Bringing Zoe Home

While Matthew and I waited anxiously at home for the arrival of the newest member of our family, Jeff began his adventure. He arrived in Moscow on May 5 and spent a day and night touring the city on his own. On May 6, Jeff met up with Dmitri and his colleague, Olga, a practicing pediatrician. Olga was to travel with Jeff and the two other families, acting as an interpreter and as liaison with the orphanage staff and local officials. Instead of risking Aeroflot, which has an even worse reputation for its domestic Russian flights than for its international routes, Jeff chose to travel by train to the city of Yoshkar-Ola. This was an eighteen-hour trip east from Moscow toward the Ural Mountains, into the heart of the Volga River valley.

Yoshkar-Ola is a small city, a cluster of ancient churches, open-air markets, light manufacturing plants, and bleak housing projects set in the flat industrial landscape of the Volga region. Jeff stayed with a young couple who had sent their daughter to stay with her grandparents in order to make space for Jeff in their tiny two-bedroom apartment. His days were spent shuttling between the orphanage and various government offices and courtrooms. At night Jeff had dinner with his new friends, phoning me as often as he could to tell me how much happier our daughter was than she looked on the video, and how she was even more beautiful. Eventually the two of them made their way back to Moscow, where their first stop was the McDonald's in Pushkin Square, where our little girl devoured two cheeseburgers and a large order of fries before falling asleep in her daddy's arms. They spent the next few days touring the city together—they even went to Lenin's tomb, which to me seemed a little too spooky for a toddler, but Jeff said the old man looked pretty good, considering—while the U.S. embassy processed our immigration paperwork. Then, May 19 arrived, and the long flight home began.

The time for me to meet Zoe had finally come. I decided that I wanted this moment for myself and to let Matthew have his own special introduction, so I went to the airport alone. There I was, standing at the arrival gate waiting to see my daughter for the first time. I looked around, thinking to myself that none of these people had any idea that they were about to witness a family being made. Wow! With tears trickling down my cheeks, I caught a glimpse of Jeff and Zoe coming into view. Jeff was pushing Zoe in a luggage cart with her only possession from the orphanage, a pacifier, in her mouth. They were a sight for sore eyes! I lifted Zoe out of the cart and carried her to the car. She seemed jet-lagged but quite content.

After we arrived home Matthew joined us to meet his little sister. When he walked into the house, I told him, "Here is your new sister," to which he quite matter-of-factly responded, "I know"—which has become a very famous statement in our home. Matthew and Zoe started playing with each other right away, and suddenly we were a brand-new family.

Due to her jet lag and unfamiliar environment, I decided to stay with Zoe in her room that first night. To my surprise, she slept all night, no problems, and I realized that this was one definite advantage of adopting an eighteen-month-old instead of an infant. Other surprises: Zoe had enough experience looking after herself that she was also able to eat with a spoon, dress herself, and put on her own shoes. It is amazing what children can learn when they have to be self-sufficient.

However, despite learning some short-term survival skills, children who spend significant time in an orphanage almost always suffer developmental delays over the long term. Even under the most comfortable and sanitary conditions, and even with the most loving caregivers, the lack of regular one-on-one attention and, in most cases, of proper nutrition has resulted in delayed development for a majority of children who spend their infancy in orphanages. When Zoe arrived home her behavior and cognitive skills were already somewhat delayed. Underweight and small for her age, she did not look like she was eighteen months old.

What we know now is that, as long as there are no other serious health problems, formerly institutionalized children will start to thrive and will grow by leaps and bounds soon after leaving the orphanage. This is why I strongly recommend that a baseline developmental evaluation be conducted as soon as possible after a child arrives home. An evaluation will allow for the child's development to be monitored for "red flags" that can signal treatable developmental issues, permitting early intervention. Another absolute must is an immediate trip to the pediatrician for a complete physical examination and blood tests for hepatitis, anemia, lead poisoning, and HIV, as well as tests for tuberculosis and parasites. Of course, most children are fine (for example, I have not heard of any children testing positive for HIV upon arrival when the adoptive parents had not already known the child was infected), but these screenings need to be done.

The day after Zoe arrived we took the poor jet-lagged little girl for a physical and a full battery of lab tests. The results were not too surprising: she was a bit anemic, suffered from poor nutrition, was small for her age, and had rickets due to a vitamin D deficiency. All of these problems have since been resolved; in fact, they were all completely gone within a few months. Zoe is now in the fiftieth percentile for height and weight, remarkably strong and well coordinated, and otherwise very healthy. It has been amazing to watch her grow. Within three months, Zoe gained three pounds and grew two inches, and by her second birthday in the November after she arrived home she had gained another three pounds and had grown another two inches. This rapid turnaround is very typical of children who are developmentally delayed as a result of poor nutrition and who have no other serious health problems.

Another very important adoption milestone is bonding and attachment. I was prepared to take things slowly and was happily surprised to see how quickly Zoe bonded with her new family. Within days she chose me over anyone else in the room—as she had chosen Jeff when they were in Russia together—because when Jeff went back to work, Zoe could see that I would be her primary caregiver, and so she came to me for comfort. A child choosing a parent over anyone else is an essential sign of attachment. Children who go from person to person and express love and affection indiscriminately may have attachment problems, and these need to be addressed by a mental health professional with experience in the behavioral issues that affect formerly institutionalized children. The longer a child has been in an orphanage, the more the child is at risk for these bonding and attachment problems.

Zoe became a part of our family so quickly that, I have to admit, she bonded with me faster than I bonded with her. For some parents, bonding with a new child comes very quickly, but for many parents this process takes time, and at first I was convinced that there must be something wrong with me. I felt as if I were baby-sitting someone else's child. I told everyone that she was adopted, even the salesperson in the shoe store. Although I cared about Zoe, she did not feel like mine.

I found, however, that bonding, even when it doesn't happen immediately, ultimately comes from shared experiences. Within a few months, my detachment was gone and Zoe felt like and truly was my daughter—and Matthew had his instant playmate and Jeff had his little princess. Finally, after the stress of my infertility experience and the long adoption process, I was able to relax.

ADOPTION AND HERITAGE

From the beginning, Jeff and I decided that we would be completely open about Zoe's adoption and not keep it a secret. My opinion has always been that family secrets are dangerous. Making adoption a taboo subject in the home sends the message that something is wrong with adoption, so we tried to weave the adoption story into the fabric of our family's everyday life. Often, I would tell Zoe the story of how she came to be with us. It became her favorite bedtime request. I also bought her several children's books that depicted adoption stories she could understand. One of the best, Keiko Kasza's (1992) *A Mother for Choco,* is about a mother bear that raises several different kinds of animals as her own children. Stories are a wonderful way to introduce and explain the concept of adoption.

May 19 has become a very special day in our home. It is the day we celebrate Brother/Sister Day, the anniversary of becoming a family. We honor this day by spending time together having family fun and, of course, a homemade cake. I believe it is very important to acknowledge birthdays as well as the adoption day. Both days are landmarks in a child's life, and both provide wonderful opportunities to discuss how a child came into the world and became part of a family.

Another principle we agreed on is that Zoe should have relationships with other adopted children and be aware of her Russian heritage. During the adoption process, I became involved with a support network of families adopting children from Eastern Europe, FRUA, which started as a small group of some forty adoptive families with children from Russia and the Ukraine. It has since grown into a national not-for-profit organization with over 2,000 members, consisting of professionals and families who have adopted children from all over Eastern Europe. My own involvement also grew until I became FRUA's chair in 1995.

I cannot stress enough how important a support network is for both parents and children. FRUA provides Zoe with a connection to other children adopted from Russia, some of whom have become her close friends. For parents, FRUA provides preadoption and postadoption information, education, and resources, and a forum for families to share their stories and helpful advice. FRUA also gives adoptive families a way to learn about the history and culture of Eastern Europe through social gatherings and special events. To learn more about FRUA, go to its Web site (www.frua.org). It is filled with preadoption and postadoption information, a chat room, resource lists, book lists, and local chapter news. Although FRUA is not an adoption agency and does not make any referrals to adoption agencies, the Web site contains plenty of information and members' views concerning the agencies currently working in Eastern Europe.

FRUA has also given my family and others the ability to help children who will never have permanent families—children spending their childhoods in institutions. FRUA has built playgrounds at Romanian orphanages and supplied needed food, vitamins, medicine, toys, and clothing to orphanages throughout Eastern Europe.

ZOE TODAY

For me, the unfolding surprise of a child growing in ways you could not have predicted is one of the wonderful things about adoption. Zoe has blossomed into a healthy, happy, and beautiful nine-year-old. She has skills and talents that I never dreamed of having myself. She is an amazing athlete and a budding artist and pianist. Never did I imagine having a daughter who would be invited to play on the girls' "travel" soccer team, representing her hometown in a regional league! Zoe has shown some delays in the development of her expressive language skills, which is common for formerly institutionalized children. She sees a language tutor twice a week, however, and is progressing well. Zoe is a very conscientious student and enjoys school. She has many friends both at school and in our neighborhood. She enjoys spending time with her peers but also enjoys quiet time alone building puzzles, reading books, and creating art.

Zoe has a very tight connection to her family. She has wonderful grandparents, aunts, uncles, and cousins who adore her and with whom she enjoys spending time. Zoe and Matthew have an incredible relationship. He has been an amazing role model for her and she has been a great friend for him. They enjoy each other's company, with the usual sibling quarrels from time to time. We have fun spending time together as a family and feel very lucky.

Zoe is beginning to ask more questions about adoption. I subscribe to the theory that a parent should answer the questions that are asked, no more, no less, because a child asks questions when he or she is ready to hear and understand the answers. Zoe knows that a man and a woman living in Russia gave her the gift of life, and that she grew in the woman's uterus. She knows that she lived in a home with many other children until she was eighteen months old, when she found a family and we found our little girl. She knows that she grew in our hearts while we waited for her to come home. If she wants to go to Russia some day, see where she was born, and look for her birth parents, I would be happy to join her on that adventure.

In today's society there are many ways that families are formed. Adoption is one of those ways. Adoption gives waiting parents a child and provides children with loving families. Dealing with infertility was a very difficult chapter in our lives. Adoption gave us hope. I am thankful for that difficult period in my life and would not want to change it. The path of infertility brought us to the path of adoption and to our daughter, Zoe, whom we adore and cherish with our hearts and souls.

REFERENCE

Kasza, K. (1992). *A mother for Choco*. New York: G.P. Putnam's Sons.

Chapter 11

Miracle Sisters from Romania

William D. Palmer

Unlike the experience of many others who have adopted, the adoption of two Romanian children into our family was not the result of some long and deliberate process, but rather the response to a call felt deep within us that such adoptions should take place.

OUR DECISION TO ADOPT

Our family was not a typical adoptive family (if there is such a thing). My wife Nancy and I both had busy legal practices. I was a partner in a large law firm and Nancy practiced family law, including adoptions and family mediation, as the head of the family law department of another large law firm. We were both in our late thirties and already had three children in our family: Brent, Nancy's son from a previous marriage, who was twelve years of age; Nicholas, my son from a prior marriage, who was also twelve; and Carley, our daughter together, who was four years old. In five years of marriage, we had never even talked about the possibility of adoption. That all changed in late 1980.

At that time, I began to feel a strong conviction that God wanted us to adopt a child from Romania. Although I was a Christian and active in my church, I had never previously felt the prompting of God to undertake a specific course of action. Recent television programs had focused on the plight of abandoned Romanian children, but neither Nancy nor I had watched them, so I had not gotten the idea from them. The crisis of abandoned children in Romania had been brought about by the policies of Communist dictator Nicolae Ceausesco, who had been overthrown and murdered, along with his wife, the previous year in the Christmas Day Massacre. Ceausesco had implemented an official state policy to encourage families to have children in order to provide soldiers for the armed forces. As a result, many families had more children then they could afford, resulting in an abundance of abandoned children residing in orphanages. The economy there had also become so poor that some Romanian families were willing to let their children be adopted by foreigners in order to receive money for food or other necessities of life.

The idea of adding another child to our already busy family and professional lives seemed to make no logical sense at all, and, accordingly, I made no mention of it to Nancy at the time. However, the thought did not go away. After several days, Nancy, out of the blue, brought up the subject with me, indicating that she had had an overwhelming conviction that a Romanian child was to come live with us. My response astounded her: "I've had the exact same thought! But it was so bizarre, I couldn't bring myself to mention it to you." As strange as the idea of adoption was at that time, the fact that simultaneously we both felt led to the same conclusion without discussion convinced us that it was God's will that we pursue such an adoption. That conviction was further strengthened when we followed up on our decision that we needed to discuss the possibility of adoption with our boys. We picked up Brent from school and told him we had something important to talk to him about. Even though the subject had never come up before, he immediately said, "If this is about adopting a child from Romania, God has already told me about it." . With such confirmation, how could we do anything but move forward?

Nancy had done private-placement adoptions but knew she would have to work with an adoption agency for an international adoption. Accordingly, she contacted Dr. Lorraine Boisselle, executive director of the Adoption Centre, Inc., to find out whether she had any knowledge about adopting from Romania. Amazingly enough, she had been to Romania within the past six months attempting to start an adoption program. However, she indicated that adoption in Romania was a great bureaucratic mess at that time and discouraged us from pursuing such an adoption. She indicated that some prospective adoptive parents had to spend weeks or months in Romania waiting for an adoption to be finalized, with no certainty that the final approval would ever come through. Nevertheless, we decided to continue to pursue this goal.

During this time frame, Dr. Boisselle called to tell us that she had a newborn American baby available for adoption and offered to place that baby with us if we wanted to adopt a little girl. We thanked her for the opportunity but declined, knowing that she would have no difficulty placing that baby with a family. On the other hand, we believed a real possibility existed that a child from Romania would remain without a family if we did not pursue such an adoption. Given the strong conviction we both had felt, we did not consider any other adoption options.

Dr. Boisselle had pictures from a recent trip to Romania and indicated that one of the children in one of the pictures might be available for adoption. She indicated the child was four years old and had health problems. Dr. Boisselle handed us a picture of two little girls. One was beautiful with a bright vivacious smile. "She's beautiful," we both said. "No," Dr. Boisselle said, pointing to the solemn, expressionless child next to her. "This is the one that may be available." It took only a day for us to pray and decide that she was the child we were supposed to adopt. Whatever the problems and hurdles, we would proceed.

Dr. Boisselle advised us that the child, whose name was Ioanna, was living in a hospital in Bucharest and had been there for two years. She originally had been admitted to the hospital with severe diarrhea and dehydration, and the hospital had diagnosed her as being allergic to wheat. Hospital personnel removed wheat products from her diet and her health returned to normal. However, her mother was unable to take care of her and so she remained in the hospital. She had become the special "pet" of the hospital ward, since she was relatively healthy and had been at the hospital for such a long time. (After she came to the United States, she repeatedly talked about "Momma Doctor" who cared for her while she was in the hospital.)

Although her mother, Cossette, had been unable to take care of her and had left her in the hospital, she indicated that she would sign a consent for adoption only if she met at least one of the prospective parents and gave her approval. Although an adoption could potentially go forward on the basis of abandonment without parental consent, a signed consent would make the process quicker and simpler. (Ioanna's father had long ago abandoned the family and his parental rights were already terminated.) Accordingly, arrangements would have to be made for one of us to travel to Romania. Potential travel was complicated by the fact that the Gulf War had just begun and the State Department was discouraging international travel. Nonetheless, we decided that Nancy would make the trip. Arrangements were made quickly for Nancy to go, along with Dr. Boisselle and another woman who had previously adopted. This family hoped to add one or two adopted Romanian children to the several children they had already adopted from other countries. Dr. Boisselle planned to pursue her desire to set up an adoption program in Romania and thought Nancy's legal and adoption experience might be helpful in that regard.

At the same time, the home study process began through the Adoption Centre, resulting in a favorable recommendation for the adoption.

We were advised that the Romanian officials were often impressed by letters of recommendation on embossed stationery, so Nancy traveled to Romania in February 1991 armed with letters of introduction and references from the mayor of Orlando, the governor of Florida, and Florida Supreme Court Justice Ben Overton, who had helped the Romanians write their new constitution. We had also been advised that Kent 100s cigarettes were invaluable for obtaining small favors in Romania, such as getting to the head of a line, finding a hotel room, obtaining an appointment, or catching a taxicab, so Nancy went laden with cartons of this valuable commodity when she left for Romania.

To make the experience particularly unique, and to document it, a local television reporter and cameraman also went on the trip, since the other family was prominent in Orlando. As a result, we were able to obtain professional videotape of Nancy's first meeting with Ioanna, Nancy meeting with Cossette, and the hospital where Ioanna was residing. The trip resulted in a series of documentaries on the local television station titled *From Romania with Love*. Our adoption experience was also detailed in a book about blended families authored by us, titled *The Family Puzzle: Putting the Pieces Together* (1996).

Dr. Boisselle had made arrangements for a local guide to be with the party throughout the ten days they were scheduled to be in Romania, to act as translator, to help in finding a Romanian attorney, and to get everyone to the places they needed to go.

Bucharest was covered in snow when the party arrived. At the airport in Bucharest, Nancy observed couples that appeared to be engaged in the buying and selling of babies, which we had previously heard about. In Bucharest, heat and hot water were available only intermittently, and hotel accommodations were limited. Shelves in shops were virtually empty. Restaurants were scarce and inevitably had menus limited to chorba (a type of beef stew) and orange soda. In one restaurant, Nancy and her party were thrilled to see a menu featuring steak, seafood, shrimp, and other delights. They soon learned, however, that the only available items were chorba and orange soda. The menus were simply left over from years earlier when such things had been available.

Upon arriving in Romania, Nancy met with Cossette, who agreed to sign consent papers to give Ioanna a better life in America. She did not ask for, or receive, any payment for executing consent forms. Although the hospital was only a fifteen-minute bus ride from Cossette's apartment, she had visited Ioanna only twice in two years and still had a Christmas present for Ioanna from her employer in her apartment. In spite of this history, she suddenly became attentive and insisted on seeing Ioanna several times before Ioanna left Romania to come to the United States. (We later learned that she had been diagnosed as clinically depressed, which undoubtedly contributed to her erratic behavior regarding contact with Ioanna.) Cossette was kind enough to provide us with baby pictures of Ioanna, including a picture of her baptism. Cossette had been a concert pianist and showed us photographs of one of her performances with the orchestra, as well as her wedding pictures. She also gave us two beautiful oil paintings done by one of Ioanna's uncles, so Ioanna would have a link to her birth family. The talent displayed in these paintings (which hang in our home today) provides a clue as to the hereditary nature of Ioanna's incredible artistic talents.

Nancy went to the hospital with small gifts for Ioanna and the hospital staff. Ioanna had been told her new mommy was coming to see her and anxiously, but quietly, crawled into Nancy's lap and began playing with her gifts.

It was then necessary to obtain an appointment with the state adoption committee in order to move forward with the adoption. With the letter of introduction from Justice Overton, Nancy was able to get in without an appointment to see the chief justice of the Romanian Supreme Court, who had worked on the drafting of the new constitution with Justice Overton. He was kind enough to make a phone call on the spot to the state adoption committee and promptly got an appointment for Nancy. The interview was held within days, the questions asked were straightforward and brief, and the adoption was promptly approved. It was also necessary to hire a Romanian attorney to finalize the adoption in Romania. At the cost of $500, Romanian counsel was secured and the legal proceedings in Romania were commenced. At this point, the Kent 100s came in handy and helped move Nancy and our attorney to the front of the line for quicker attention. After fewer than ten days in Romania, Nancy was able to attend a final adoption hearing and return to the United States with a Romanian adoption decree in hand and promises that Ioanna could join us in a matter of weeks, once immigration paperwork was completed by the U.S. Embassy.

Nancy returned home with videos and photographs of Ioanna but with the inevitable fear of what might happen if something prevented the immigration paperwork from being completed. My eyes filled with tears when I viewed the videotape of Nancy's first meeting with our new daughter, even though I had not yet met her. Carley did her part to speed up her new sister's arrival in the United States. At a mother-daughter tea held at our church in early May, she slipped onto the stage without the prompting or knowledge of Nancy and asked the assembled crowd to pray that her sister from Romania would be able to join the family without any problems. In fact, no glitches occurred and immigration approval was given the following week. I was scheduled to return to Romania to pick up Ioanna, but my friend had moved forward on the adoption of two Romanian children and was able to bring Ioanna home along with one of her new daughters. On the night before Mother's Day (May 13, 1991), Ioanna arrived at Orlando International Airport to meet her new family.

We completed the legal adoption process in Romania on February 28, one day before they placed a moratorium on further adoption finalizations, and Ioanna came to the United States two weeks before Romania imposed a moratorium on further adoptive children leaving the country pending the implementation of new adoption policies. These facts further confirmed our belief that this adoption was meant to occur, and exactly when it did.

Dr. Boisselle graciously handled the entire process for only a few thousand dollars, much less than her usual adoption fees, in light of the personal relationship we shared with her and the legal expertise Nancy had provided to her. Unfortunately, in light of the moratorium and subsequent restrictions imposed on adoptions, Dr. Boisselle was never able to start an adoption program in Romania.

When Ioanna arrived, we promptly changed her name to Joanna, providing her with a more American name without having to change her original name very much. We changed her middle name to Marin, her birth mother's maiden name, to maintain a tie for her with her Romanian roots. She spoke no English when she arrived, and our Romanian language skills were limited to a list of one hundred words that had been provided to us. We did find a local person who spoke Romanian and was kind enough to come to the house the first weekend to explain to Joanna who her new family was and to show her around her new home.

One of the great highlights, from Joanna's standpoint, of her initial weekend in America was shoes. She had apparently never had a real pair of shoes, having lived in hospital slippers for the previous two years. She immediately put on a pair of shoes and for three days would not take them off. She slept in them, swam in them, and took her bath in them. Eventually she adjusted to the idea that the shoes would still be there for her after she took them off, and so she would then do so.

Her arrival required adjustments by the whole family. The abuse or neglect she had suffered became evident. She hit and bit herself, she screamed and spit at us, and she would vigorously rock herself to sleep at night. However, with wonderful help from counselors and others, she adjusted and adapted wonderfully to her new family. The Jewish Community Center (JCC) played a vital role in this adjustment. Its preschool program was generally considered one of the best in the area and our son, Brent, had attended many years earlier. In spite of Joanna's history, behaviors, and lack of English skills, the JCC welcomed her with open arms, lavished love and attention upon her, and helped her become a happy, well-adjusted child. Her classmates readily accepted her both here and at other schools later, further helping with the adjustment.

Although we had been told she was likely borderline mentally retarded, we soon learned that Romania had trouble properly administering intelligence tests, and she was actually gifted. In spite of coming to America with no knowledge of the English language, within two months she spoke English fluently.

We made the conscious decision not to cultivate or promote her proficiency in speaking Romanian. After Joanna had been here for a few weeks, we attended a picnic of families who had adopted Romanian children. Several people at the picnic were speaking Romanian and Joanna reacted very negatively to it, running away in apparent terror. We decided she had so many negative feelings associated with her time in Romania that a clean break was preferable. In our situation, that decision seems to have served us well.

In light of the earlier diagnosis of wheat allergy, we kept her off all wheat products for a few months. However, at our pediatrician's suggestion, we slowly introduced wheat products and discovered she had no allergy at all. Either she had outgrown her allergy, had been miraculously healed, or had been incorrectly diagnosed in Romania. (We had learned that medical practices in Romania were very out of date, since no medical class had graduated in the country since the 1940s. When Joanna had first arrived, she came with pills from the hospital that we were told it was critical she take. We quickly determined that the pills were simply saccharin, which has no medical value.)

As soon as Joanna was eligible (six months after arrival), we applied to make her a U.S. citizen. Within only a couple of months, the paperwork was completed and she received her citizenship.

We also filed legal papers in Florida to readopt Joanna. Although a Florida adoption was not technically required in light of the adoption finalization in Romania, we thought a Florida adoption decree, in English, would be more helpful when seeking such things as a Social Security number or school admission than a decree in Romanian, which would need to be translated. We felt the process was well worth undertaking and regularly recommended it to our clients who had finalized adoptions in foreign countries.

Adjustments over time were required. Nicholas remembers that when Joanna first came she spit at him and threw things and broke things in the house. Such conduct is not easy for an adolescent to watch. Yet, over time, the two of them really tightened their relationship. Joanna liked to point out how her skin was brown like Nicholas's; this gave her a physical connection she could see and touch.

I remember several notable adjustment issues. The first time the shower was put on Joanna, she screamed horribly. We concluded she must have been burned once in the shower and was reacting accordingly. The first Fourth of July she spent with us we attended a fireworks show. When the first fireworks went off, she trembled and hid under her seat. She later explained, "When we heard those sounds in the hospital, they moved us all down into the basement." She obviously had memories from the revolution that had toppled the Romanian dictator. After Joanna had been here approximately a year, we raised the possibility that we might sell the house we were in and move to another house. Joanna became visibly sad and struggled to fight back tears. She then asked us the important question that was on her mind: "If we leave this house, can we take the food with us?" Being without food seemed to be a continuation of fears she had had when she first arrived and would hide some of her food without eating it.

Shortly after her arrival, a simple scrape on her knee became badly infected, requiring a trip to the doctor. We learned on that trip that Joanna was more susceptible to infection than children born here because she was being exposed to germs different from those she had been exposed to in Romania. We also learned on that trip of her great fear of doctors and shots, which continues to this day, probably resulting from her early experiences in the hospital. Such fear extends to trips to the dentist as well, where she will shake continuously from arrival to departure. Overall, however, her adjustment has been remarkable. She is now fifteen years old and a beautiful, well-adjusted young lady. She attends an engineering and technology magnet program at a local high school, where she carries better than a 3.5 grade point average. She is a talented artist and a gifted chef. In fact, she has already settled on a career plan to go to culinary school, become a chef, and ultimately own her own restaurant.

Joanna's relationship with her sister Carley has gone through periods of closeness and periods not so close, as with most sisters. Carley had to go from being the only girl (and the baby) in the family to sharing attention with a slightly younger sister. Although the girls are only 100 days apart in age, we started Carley in school a year early, resulting in the girls being in different grades. We found the difference in grades to be a distinct advantage, since the competition and comparisons that would inevitably have existed between them if they were in the same classes were avoided. In fact, for much of their schooling, they ended up not only in different grades but also in different schools, reducing even further the chances for competitiveness and comparisons. We always tried to select schools based on our children's individual needs and talents (at one time resulting in having five children in five different schools) and determined at one point that Carley was better suited to public school while Joanna was better suited to a church school. Now they attend different high schools, since Carley is in a special magnet program in a school outside of our district in order to earn an international baccalaureate degree.

Nick bonded more quickly and closely with Joanna than did Brent, who seemed to develop more affinity and bonding with Carley. The boys are now both going to law school and live together in Gainesville, so their time with either girl is significantly limited. However, it is fair to say that both willingly accepted Joanna into the family and considered her as much a part of the family as any other member.

JOANNA'S HALF SISTER ARRIVES

Five years later, we repeated the adoption experience (with several distinct twists and differences) with Joanna's half sister, Mihaela, who was fifteen at the time. We had maintained some written contact with Cossette through the years, keeping her updated on Joanna's progress and successes. She then contacted us to ask if we would be willing to adopt Mihaela, who had been living on and off with her and with Cossette's parents, in order to give her a chance at a better life than she could have in Romania. We promptly said yes, believing that uniting her with her sister would be beneficial for all. Mihaela knew a fair amount of English, having studied it for four years in school, so she was able to write letters to us from Romania expressing her desire to come to the United States. However, we were advised that, given her age and the state of immigration law at the time, we would not be able to adopt her since she had not lived with us outside of the country for at least a year. Undeterred, we looked into other available options. The option that seemed best was to bring Mihaela to this country on a student visa, which we were able to obtain through the local public high school in a matter of weeks, without the necessity of a trip to Romania. In January of 1995, Cossette put her on a plane in Romania and she flew unaccompanied to the United States to begin her new life with us.

Mihaela quickly adapted to American life. She had had access to MTV in Romania, so her exposure to American music and culture was greater than we had expected. However, when we took her out for fast food after picking her up from the airport, we learned that she had never been in a restaurant before.

After her first day in school, she came home and announced that she had changed her name to Michelle, since Mihaela was too difficult for people to pronounce. (Two years later, she would return to using the name Mihaela, appreciating its uniqueness and exotic sound.)

In many ways, Mihaela's adjustment to a new family and a new country were tougher than Joanna's, since she started at the age of fifteen years. Initially Mihaela seemed to bond more closely with Carley, with whom she had no blood tie, than with Joanna. Over time, however, her bonds with both girls have fluctuated in strength, as with those among all of our children over time.

For two sixteen-year-old boys, adding a fifteen-year-old girl to the family was far different from adding a four-year-old when they were twelve. Although they may have thought we were crazy to add another child to our hectic life, they did their best to introduce her to American life. However, since they both went to high schools outside of our district, she was in a different school from them and had to fit into her new school without their help. In addition, since each boy spent a significant amount of time with his other parent, neither was at the house full-time to help.

We dealt with many adjustment problems with Mihaela, including experimentation with alcohol and starting out with the wrong crowd of friends. When she took the family car without permission and without a driver's license to go visit a boyfriend (taking Joanna in the car with her and leaving Carley home alone because she refused to get into the car), we came close to sending her back to Romania. Having not yet adopted her, we felt that option was still available to us and frankly told her that, although we loved her dearly, we would not allow her to endanger Joanna and the rest of our family. Talking to her as strongly as we did had its effect, and after an extended period of grounding, the problems did not reoccur. We recognize that, to some extent, the problems we experienced with her are ones experienced by many people with a daughter going through adolescence, and not necessarily tied to her relocation to a new family and a new country, though undoubtedly those factors played a part. Fortunately, Nancy and I have a strong marriage and a strong faith, which have helped us weather the difficult times with all of our children without weakening our love or our marriage.

Mihaela has retained her ties to Romania and the Romanian language far more than Joanna, as would be expected in light of her fifteen years there. She has maintained regular telephone contact with both her birth mother and her grandparents in Romania, together with written contact. Although a little rusty, her Romanian language skills remain usable. She has acted as translator to make it possible for Joanna to talk to her birth mother and grandparents, since they know no English and Joanna retains no Romanian. Joanna's aversion to hearing Romanian spoken has now disappeared, and she has asked Mihaela to reteach her the language.

Since Mihaela came to the United States on a student visa, the adoption issue was more complicated than with Joanna. As she had lived intermittently with her mother and grandparents in Romania, she technically was not abandoned and, therefore, was not available for adoption in Romania. Having arrived in the United States on a student visa, she also did not qualify for adoption as a minor in the United States. However, once she reached the age of majority, she could consent to an adoption on her own and we could proceed forward with an adult adoption. As a result, as of October 2000, Mihaela legally became our daughter through formal adult adoption proceedings. Unfortunately, being adopted as an adult did not alter her immigration status, so she remains in the country pursuant to the student visa originally issued to her. As long as she remains in school on a full-time basis, her visa remains valid. Once she completes school, however, she will need to find another way to stay in the country, perhaps through a special work visa, a green card, or by falling in love with and marrying an American. Since she is currently completing work on her bachelor's degree and hopes ultimately to get a doctoral degree in Christian counseling, she has many more years of eligibility on a student visa before she will have to work out other arrangements to stay in the country.

Mihaela's entry into the family on a student visa created a few issues of disparate conduct toward different children that we had to address. For example, we generally do not supply cars to our children because they can get jobs and earn money if they want cars. Mihaela does not have that option because she is ineligible to work while in the country on a student visa. Similarly, other luxuries that the other children can buy with money earned on jobs are not available to Mihaela in the same way. Instead she might have to do more jobs around the house in exchange for such things. Although having to apply different rules to different children creates some challenges, these challenges are not insurmountable.

As we have advised others in *The Family Puzzle,* we tried always to remember that when difficulties arose, we should not assume that they were the result of the girls' background or the adoptions but just as likely were difficulties that arise in the raising of any children.

In spite of the adjustment and immigration difficulties we have faced, the joys have far outnumbered the difficulties, and we would absolutely repeat the experience if we had it to do over again. Although we recognize that adoption is not for everyone, when God called on us, we could do nothing but listen and follow his direction.

REFERENCE

Palmer, Nancy S. and Palmer, William D., with Kay Marshall Strom (1996). *The family puzzle: Putting the pieces together, a guide to parenting the blended family.* Colorado Springs, CO: Pinon Press.

Chapter 12

Adventures in Adoption: From Russia to America

Anne

We were not going to adopt again . . . had no intention of it. Then a little boy literally landed on our doorstep . . .

Our adventure with adoption was very much like our adventure in marriage: one of us saying, "Hey, that is a great idea," and the other thinking, "This is a lifelong commitment; suppose I don't like it?" I usually make decisions more quickly than my husband does, figuring that somehow I will be able to juggle whatever I have to juggle as it comes along. It is a method that can be chaotic, but it works for me. My husband, Dave, likes to study issues and know all the angles before venturing into serious decisions. On the other hand, when we go to the beach, he is the first in the water, and once he learned how to negotiate moguls, he was not afraid to ski down a steep slope.

We married late in life. I was forty-four, he was forty-five. He was definitely worth the wait. Neither of us had had children, and when we got married, we decided we would not do anything to prevent pregnancy. Nearly two years later, I still was not pregnant, so we did the usual tests and then talked to my gynecologist, who discussed probability and cost versus benefit, with the warning that infertility treatment could take over our lives and was emotionally draining, but that was not to say it could not be done. The analysis of numbers, the cost of infertility treatment versus the probability of getting pregnant, was a part of the discussion that I had not expected. I, the one with the degree in drama, decided the numbers did not add up. My husband,

---

This chapter is written under a pseudonym, and with family members' names changed to protect their identities and privacy.

the numbers guy, decided it was emotionally too difficult to see me so ill after having general anesthesia.

I mourned my infertility for half an hour, maybe half a day. It did not take long to decide that my life could be complete without ever being pregnant. It just would not be complete without having a child of my own. I wanted a little girl.

THE PREADOPTION PHASE

"I never wanted to adopt so active a child, but I love her the way she is," said an adoptive mother at one of the adoption meetings we attended. I could not see how this child was not driving the mother nuts. She was all over the place, pulling books from the shelves, running across the room, and scattering toys. Half an hour of this with her, I thought, would make me put a gun to my head and pull the trigger. At that time I did not appreciate how much you accept as a parent. At these meetings, the parents passed around photo albums of their precious babies. They talked about the $20,000 to $30,000 it cost to adopt as if it were the same as buying a bag of sugar at the grocery store, as if that was what you should expect to pay when adopting from a country where the average salary might be twenty to forty dollars a month or maybe even less. I found the adoption industry distasteful and decided to do it on my own.

I signed us up for seminars and meetings so we could get information about building our family. Sadly, they gave us very little information. All they talked about were babies, and I was not interested in adopting a baby. I did not want to parent teenagers as a senior citizen. I did not want to be up all night with a colicky baby and then go to work the next day. I did not want to face the dilemmas my friends with babies faced when they had to find child care. Work was a reality. I did not want to look as tired as my friends with preschoolers looked when they came to work. Absolutely no one at these seminars ever spoke about eight-year-olds. I wanted a little girl between eight and ten, or seven and eleven, years of age. Six would be okay, and maybe twelve. I was flexible about the age. I just did not want a baby.

I also began networking. I spoke to adoptive mothers. Some were Caucasian women like me who adopted black babies or Hispanic babies or mixed-race babies. Sometimes it was intentional. Sometimes it "just happened." With adoption, as with any birth, some things are not totally predictable.

I also read. Some of the things you read about are scary: children who have been neglected for so long they will never be normal, children who constantly rock, children with all sorts of medical and emotional conditions. People wrote with great compassion about these children, and the people who adopted them were devoted to their care. There were also stories of disrupted adoptions and emotionally and financially exhausted and deeply disappointed parents.

I decided I wanted us to blend in as a family. I did not want strangers talking to me in the supermarket, asking all sorts of personal questions about my children or my husband. I did not know that even if I adopted Caucasian children we wouldn't blend in. Physically, we did, but my children speak Russian and I do not. I did not know I would meet people everywhere I went who spoke Russian and that I would enjoy meeting them so much.

Word got out in the Russian community in Washington, DC, that I was looking to adopt. (I worked with a lot of Russian Americans so it did not take long.) My husband was not sure he could deal with a communication gap. Could we not adopt an American or Irish child? A cousin in Ireland researched our prospects there while the county social worker offered discouraging news about American children. She explained that, unless we were willing to devote ourselves to raising an emotionally disturbed child, we would be better off looking elsewhere. The Irish cousin reported back that Irish orphans were scarce and preference was given to Irish citizens. Russia seemed to be the country with the most navigable bureaucracy and the largest number of available children.

My connections with the Russian-American community led me to the wife of an Orthodox priest who ran an orphanage near Moscow. We exchanged letters. She told me about a girl who might work out. All we had to do was spend some time in Russia to meet the girl, and if we decided to proceed she would help us with the paperwork. This sounded great! I would at last get my little girl. She tried to send me pictures, but they got lost in the mail. I told my husband, "Dave, all we have to do is go to Russia. She has even offered to translate the documents for us. A woman nearby adopted two boys from her orphanage. We could have our child in just a few months." My wonderful husband, however, could not adopt a child he did not know. This was a setback I did not know how to overcome. Adoption was put on the back burner.

Fortunately, no one else knew that but me. One summer day, I got a call from an Orthodox priest who told me about a pool party for Russian orphans visiting the United States. Never mind that it was in upstate New York, about an eight-hour drive from our home in Virginia. Dave seemed happy to go. We decided to leave early Saturday morning and get there before the party ended.

In theory, that sounded good. We were supposed to leave by 8 a.m. but pulled out of the driveway two hours later instead. Dave forgot something and we had to go back. The directions were convoluted. Dave decided to ditch them, which made me more anxious. I completely lost it when he told me we needed gas, we were lost, and the party was ending. I do not cry a lot, but I cried so hard then that I used all the tissues in the car. Dave got scared enough to ask for directions at a convenience store. You could call it fate or divine providence or synchronicity, but a man who pulled up next to us at the store was going in that direction. "Follow me," he said. He led us down an unmarked country lane that we would never have found on our own and directly to the pool party, where we got the chance to talk to the people who had hosted these children. It turned out that all fourteen of them were spoken for.

These fourteen children were the first Bridge of Hope group, a program run by the Cradle of Hope Adoption Agency in Silver Spring, Maryland. They were planning another program the following summer (1998), maybe in Washington, DC. The program's aim is to bring older Russian orphans to the United States to attend summer camp. These children are considered too old to be adopted by most Russians, and probably by most Americans, but while they are here, most of them find people who want to parent them, thus beginning their journeys toward adoption. My husband liked the idea that these children were screened and selected by the agency's staff in Russia and by the orphanage directors. They were the best of the best, the most likely to succeed. We did not know that screening can go only so far, that children react far differently in an orphanage than they do outside an institution.

The next spring, we signed up to host children in the summer of 1998. We said we would take a sibling group and that one of them had to be a girl. I was afraid if we were not open to siblings, we might end up with none. The agency requested a photo, so I used one taken while we were on a ski vacation. We had posed with our skis, and my goggles were on top of my hat. Figuring the photo would just end up in some file folder, I copied it on a black-and-white copier and handed it in. I never thought it would be first picture of us our children would see.

Then the call came. Leslie Nelson, the agency's director of social services, told me, "I have selected two girls for you. They are sisters. Marianna is ten and it says she likes to keep things in order and she makes friends easily. Katya is eight and she has dazzling energy. She's very cute. Should I fax their pictures and information to you?" Before Leslie hung up, I said, "We'll take them!" When I got the color photos provided by the director of their orphanage, I saw that both girls sported enormous red bows. Katya beamed. Marianna looked sad. My next thought was, I better tell my husband. Much to my surprise, he was delighted. Two meant they would have each other as playmates and we would have to do this only once.

In late June we drove to the agency office in Silver Spring, Maryland. As we got off the elevator, I told Dave, "When we walk through that door, our lives may change forever." I did not feel I had to adopt these children. One of my friends, an attorney who has handled adoptions, told me to approach this coolly. Evaluate them. "This will be your life," he said, "and you want to make sure you want these children to be part of it." I thought I could observe their behavior better because I did not speak Russian. I would see how they acted with each other. I even dressed up a little to make a good first impression. I did not know they had been given that strange picture of us on the ski slope. Marianna came over and hugged me. Katya examined everything in the office. They looked a little bedraggled, as anyone would after traveling for two days. Marianna wore a dress. She had wanted to make a good impression too.

"Tell them just to say 'toilet' when they need to go to the bathroom," we told our interpreter. Before taking off with our two young houseguests, we ironed out as many essentials as we could through the interpreter. We showed them pictures of our house so they would know where they were to live, a picture of our cat Dolly, and a picture of Tyotya (Aunt) Ira, a friend I work with who offered to call every day and act as an interpreter. The Russians have a nice way of making adults familiar while still including an honorific that is not as formal as the English mister or missus. Any friend of the family becomes aunt or uncle, whereas Americans reserve aunt or uncle for blood relatives. Come to think of it, Ira's picture was strange too. I had snapped a picture of her in white Minnie Mouse bridal ears while we were at Disney World in Orlando on business.

Marianna gasped when she saw our house, a four-bedroom Dutch colonial. She conveyed the feeling that this was a palace. My mother had gone shopping for me so they would have enough shorts and shirts for camp. I called my mother and father, who came over for dinner. Katya was so excited she did somersaults all the way down the hall. When she smiled, we could see that one of her front teeth was coming in. When it was time for bed, they decided they wanted to sleep in the same twin bed, and they were small enough to fit.

That summer was like a courtship. Communicating my needs was often frustrating, and I never made it to work on time, but I had planned to work shorter days so I could get to know the children. We went swimming every night and ate lots of watermelon, chicken, cucumbers, and tomatoes. By the fourth day, the girls and I knew we were a family. That evening, Marianna indicated that she wanted some paper and something to write with. I gave her markers, thinking she wanted to draw. Instead she wrote four sentences in Russian, using different colored markers. The last sentence had all our names in it. Marianna and Mama, Papa, and Katya. I asked her if I could show it to my friend Ira, and she agreed. The next day Ira read it and translated, "Marianna and Mama, Papa, and Katya are a family."

Dave, however, was not sure. He wanted more time. Our home study was done, but I could not start working on the paperwork until he gave the go-ahead. I did not know then that he would not have been able to send them back to face a life without a family. He was concerned about Katya's emotional outbursts. I was not, figuring they were due to our inability to communicate with each other. I was concerned about Marianna. There was something mysterious, something deep, about her, whereas Dave thought Marianna was the clear draw.

The last night they were here was the most horrible night of my life. By this time we had decided to adopt, yet I knew when I put them back on the bus to the airport that I had no legal hold over them. I traced their feet on paper so I would know what size shoes to buy them for their return to America, I drew hearts for toenails, and I could not stop crying. They cried too. No one got much sleep that night. Dave got up early and made them their favorite breakfast: hard-boiled eggs and home fries. Marianna still loves home fries. We told them to eat even if they were not hungry because they had a long journey ahead of them. Then we all got in my old car and drove to the adoption agency. I cried intermittently. While we waited for everyone to get there, Katya clung to me. Marianna just looked resigned. When the bus pulled away, any tears I had held back came forth. I did not know I had such an abundant supply. I still cry today when I think about that moment.

Life without Katya and Marianna was sad. For a long time, I could not go into their room, which we had filled with stuffed animals and balloons from their good-bye dinner at my mother's house. They took their Barbies, some photos, and some stuffed animals with them in their little backpacks. I filled the time by working on the seemingly endless paperwork and by scouring the house for gifts we could take to Russia with us, such as perfumes I had never opened or bath mats I had bought but did not use. I could not talk about my two girls a world away, maybe never to be mine. We read stories on the Internet about the fall of the ruble, fighting in Chechnya, and the wobbly regime of Boris Yeltsin, all things that could impact foreign adoptions.

We formed our own little support group with other waiting families. My paperwork was in by late August. Then the courts closed down for two months. I began wondering how I would live my life without them. Dave said we would quit our jobs, sell everything, and move to Russia to be near them.

Then the call came. We had a court date. We would be there for Thanksgiving and for our fifth wedding anniversary. We were going to fly Aeroflot. I started studying Russian again, although I did it with phonetic English. My eyes still crossed when I looked at Cyrillic.

When we got to the southern Russian city where our court hearing would take place, it was drizzling, though noticeably warmer than Moscow and not much different from home. We stood at the end of the runway for about an hour with our six bags of luggage and the computer printer we were ferrying from Moscow for the coordinator. We had a duffel bag of gifts for the children at the orphanage and another duffel bag of gifts for the caretakers, the orphanage director, our translator, and the regional coordinator. My shopping at home unearthed some amazing stuff, plus Dave's cousins got into the act, and there we were: Americans in a strange city, unable to speak the language, and unable to call anyone because we lacked a phone card (purchased at the post office or from some kiosk).

We took a cab to the town's hotel. Our driver was an Armenian who sang and practically danced while driving when I asked if he was Turkish. I breathed a sigh of relief when we got to the hotel. I half expected the driver to pull off on some country road and murder us. By this time, it was around midnight. We called Moscow. Who was supposed to meet us? And where should we go now? Olga, our coordinator, was in an auto accident and totaled her car that evening. Fortunately, she was not injured, nor was her son, the driver.

The next day we went to see the girls. They lived an hour away at an orphanage that seemed to have been converted from a school. Marianna looked sad. I found out they had told her we were coming the day before. She had waited and waited . . . and then we did not show up. Both girls looked strange rather than familiar. I did not see the happy faces I had in my photographs from the previous summer. Marianna had a cold sore and her blonde hair was shaggy. Katya wore big puffy bows. Both seemed distant, but it had been four months since we had seen them and there had been no communication in the meantime. I did not want to overwhelm them, so I did not attempt to kiss them or even hug them. Later, I found out they were severely disappointed.

We met in a room with a large conference table. The room seemed cavernous. Dave and I sat in chairs that lined the walls. Marianna was called to the table to write something. She began to cry. Our translator . explained that Marianna had to sign documents saying she agreed to the adoption and that she had made a mistake in signing her name. She thought the mistake meant she wouldn't be able to be adopted.

I did not sleep that night before our court hearing. I had heard stories of judges and prosecutors who opposed international adoptions and worried that we might meet up with someone like that. Then the prosecutor asked me why I wanted these girls and not some others. My eyes burned and I said it would be unthinkable. I had with me a small photo album containing pictures of the girls taken with my family the summer before. Olga told me to show it to the prosecutor. He looked at the pictures and said the girls clearly belonged with us. The judge agreed. It was over. We were parents. I remember feeling happy and dazed and awfully tired.

THE ADOPTION IS FINALIZED

Adoption, they say, is only the beginning of your journey together, not the end. At long last the girls were legally ours and the worries of never seeing them again were over. Now, however, we had children with whom we could not communicate. I had all sorts of bilingual dictionaries and phrase books, and I had purchased Russian language tapes, but I did not need to ask where there was a hairdresser or how to hail a taxi. Marianna was disappointed that I had not learned Russian in the four months since I last saw her. I should have worked harder on it, but I felt the same despairing attitude about learning Russian that they felt about English.

On the flight home, I started reading the court documents about the termination of their mother's rights and their treatment in their biological home. The write-up was chilling, but it turned out the documents were not even close to the horrors of their reality. My poor little girls had been starved and beaten. Their mother was an alcoholic and a drug abuser. She was sometimes beaten by her lovers. Sometimes they beat Marianna. There were knife fights and rapes. They were desperately poor. Sometimes they spent the entire night outdoors and no one knew where they were. Sometimes Katya had spent the night outside by herself, and she must have been only three or four years old. I did not know that the children had received almost no education. I did not know that Marianna had a severe learning disability nor how badly this poor little girl had been traumatized.

I would say our first six months together as a family were sheer hell. I apologized to my husband for ruining our lives. All four of us were terribly sleep deprived. The children could not fall asleep because they were too scared, so there would be tears and doors slamming and screaming up until midnight each night. Then it would subside and Dave and I could grab four or five hours of sleep. School was also stressful for them. The teachers would ask what to do when Marianna banged her head on the floor. They explained that Katya just grunted and made little noises as her way of communicating. At home, Marianna became violent. None of the professionals was able to help—not the teachers, nor the pediatrician, nor the therapist I consulted to manage their behavior while I searched for a Russian-speaking therapist who could help them. Dave's health started to fail: his diverticulitis became chronic and he suffered repeated infections and high fevers.

Marianna began attacking me. It happened when we were alone, which was every day after school. About a month after coming home, she threatened to hit me with a wine bottle. I was terrified but decided to ignore her and she put the bottle down. After the baby-sitters left when I got home, she would start in. She would hit me as hard as she could. She would scream obscenities at me in Russian. She punched me in the head while I was driving more than once. She bit me so hard that she would break the skin on my arms and leave terrible bruises. Once, during our tussles, she kicked me in the face. A friend taught me how to put her in a body hold. Sometimes I had to pin her to the floor for up to an hour before my husband got home and I could get away.

Friends gave us the name of a Russian-speaking child psychologist. The violence did not stop, but at least she was getting help. It was then that I learned about the horrible beatings she had suffered, and the knife wounds and cigarette burns. I tried to surround our children with friends and family. Marianna was wonderful with babies and loved little children, and when she was with other people, I could see how kind and good she was. When she was asleep, I would look at her beautiful face, her childlike hands, her thick golden hair and wonder how anyone could have hurt her as they did. Once, while I was driving in the car with her and we were alone, she told me, "No one in Russia loved me the way you love me."

Katya, meanwhile, became the little girl I had always wanted—tender, energetic, feisty, and fun. I had never thought I wanted a feisty little girl, but she was perfect. She was the light of our lives, and it was hard not to show a preference.

At a family dinner one October, Marianna began acting up. By this time we could communicate. I told her if she could not be pleasant, she'd have to take a time-out in her room. She agreed instantly, and I knew I was in for it. When we got to the top of the stairs, she started slugging. I forced her down on her bed and began taking off her shoes. That is when she kicked me with all of her might. Her heel squarely hit my cheekbone and my eye socket. I was afraid because her behavior had no boundaries. The pediatrician was concerned because she had no remorse. By this time, I was not seeing any improvement in her behavior and I was becoming increasingly worried about being maimed. Our pediatrician was now doing research on post-institutionalized children. She placed Marianna on Depakote, a drug that took the edge off her anger. I still had to put her in body holds, but she was much more manageable. It took ten months of my living in danger to get her properly medicated.

A few months later, Marianna sat at the foot of my bed and cried for three hours. She then told me that when she did this in Russia, her caretakers would send her to the hospital, where she'd get a shot in her bottom. She begged me to do something. All I had was Tylenol PM. I gave her one and hugged her and vowed that I would find a way to help her. Despite everything, I loved her. Her behavior with other people was so good that it was off the scale. Her behavior with me and my sister-in-law was dangerous. On top of that, she was often sullen, angry, and vile. All the hatred and anger she felt for the way she had been treated in Russia was directed at me, and there was no sign she was improving. I felt like I lived with Linda Blair's character in *The Exorcist.*

I finally got an appointment with a psychopharmacologist at Children's Hospital. It took two months from the time I called to book an appointment. Dr. Joshi, chief of child psychiatry at the hospital, informed me she could not evaluate Marianna on an outpatient basis. She had to be admitted. Marianna actually looked forward to it. She thought she would learn how to control her temper. Plus, it was a break from living with me. I looked forward to it too. The day we took Marianna to the hospital, we took Katya out to dinner. She wanted to go out like a regular family, not a family with a problem child. We went to a simple, family-style restaurant and had a wonderful time. To think that this is what it could be like . . .

Ten days without Marianna, I thought, would be bliss, but that was not how it was to be. Dave said he did not want Marianna to feel abandoned and we were going to visit her every day. So the three I had envisioned to be together were a different three, and we had to find a baby-sitter for Katya because the hospital was so far away from our house that we never made it home before 9 p.m. or, more often, 10 p.m. Marianna was delighted with our visits, especially the night I went to visit her alone. Her being admitted to the hospital was the best thing that could have happened. We learned a lot about her, and she learned a lot too. She thought we had adopted her because she was blonde. In fact, we adopted her because she was kind and generous. I think finding that out surprised her. It took me a couple of years to figure out how she formed that opinion: five children from her orphanage participated in the Bridge of Hope program, and the three who did not get adopted had brown hair.

At Children's Hospital, tests showed Marianna had a significant central auditory processing disability. The doctors impressed upon us how difficult it was for her to learn English. We also found out more about the abuse in her background. Her diagnosis: post-traumatic stress disorder. We had a survivor of seven years of torture. She was starting to talk about her past, and just when we thought we had heard the worst of it, she would tell me something else that made my blood run cold. Fortunately, a brain scan showed no physical brain damage from the abuse.

As the days edged closer to Marianna's return, I began to feel that I could not do it any longer. I began making calls to see where else I could place her. I doubted anyone would adopt her. By this time, she was nearly twelve. Again, Dave stepped in and vetoed the idea. "She's been flushed down the toilet by everyone she's ever known," he said, "and we're not doing it to her. Besides, we don't know how it would affect Katya. Maybe she'd get the idea that she's next." Dave and Katya had formed their own mutual admiration society. She worshiped the ground he walked on. Her kindness, and especially her concern for him when he was sick, touched his heart.

There is a term social workers use when you accept a child unconditionally. They say that you "claim" that child, meaning you have accepted that child as part of your family no matter what. I did not know of the term at the time, but it was at that point we claimed Marianna. She had brought up the idea of joining a different family. We told her there would be no other family, even if she did not like us sometimes. This was the spring of 2000. We had been a family for a year and a half.

As the days went by, I began seeing subtle improvements in Marianna's behavior. She was not hitting as often, and her recovery periods were becoming shorter. Usually after a fight we would feel distant for a week or two; now the time was lessening. It was frightening for her to trust someone. A wonderful evening during which she and I would read stories and talk would always be followed the next day by an explosion. Getting close was scary and she had to back away.

That spring, Dave had major surgery. He had gotten so ill, I was afraid of losing him. The surgery was a huge success and he has not been bothered by diverticulitis since. I no longer had to take the girls away on weekends and keep them away from home as long as possible so he could rest. He was able to help me more with the children. He and Katya continued to develop their own sphere of love. Marianna continued to be difficult, but one day she announced that Papa was the best breakfast maker ever, and she began in a very small way to develop a relationship with him.

By the following summer, I was researching boarding schools for Marianna. She was so oppositional and verbally abusive that I felt I could not live with her anymore, but I did not want her to be far away. I wanted her to be able to come home on the weekends, to still be a part of the family, and I wanted a school that would address her learning disability.

The week of July 4, she had no summer camp. My husband was to drive her to his sister's house on the New Jersey shore. Usually, when Dave and Marianna were together, there was total silence. This time, she chatted nonstop. My sister-in-law reported a change in her behavior too. She was still exhausting to be with, but she did not lose her temper even once during that visit and she was more compliant.

Something happened that summer. Maybe she finally figured out that we had claimed her. When she returned home, her good behavior continued. Then the call came. "Would you be able to take a little boy in your house for just a few days? He's going back to Russia early, and we need someplace to put him." It was Linda Perilstein, director of Cradle of Hope. Peter was a Bridge of Hope camper who had not worked out in his initial home. Sending a child back early was highly unusual. His host mother was convinced he was emotionally disturbed. I could not take the next day off from work, but I knew that sending him back would end any chance he had of being adopted. If we could find him a camp, maybe he could stay with us. I called my husband and asked what he thought about having a seven-year-old boy stay with us for three weeks. I found a camp for him at Katya's school.

PETER ENTERS OUR HEARTS
AND OUR FAMILY

Back on the phone with Linda, I asked, "What was he doing that was so awful that he was going home early?" The behaviors she described were ones I felt I could handle. Besides, three weeks of hell lasts only three weeks; there is an end to it. I knew what hell was. He was not hurling lamps or furniture at people and he was not clobbering anyone. My behavior standards were met. That weekend, when Dave went to pick up Peter from his interim home, he found a little boy with dark hair and green eyes like mine and a face splashed with freckles. When Peter saw Dave, the little boy started to cry, his forty-two-pound frame heaving with sobs.

"Mom, I want a little brother, I want a little brother, I want a little brother. What did I just say?" Marianna asked when I told her a little boy would be staying with us. Ever since Marianna could talk to me, she asked, "Why did you adopt two? Why not one?" One day I told her, "Because there were two of you. If there were three I would have adopted three." It was then that she offered, "There used to be three." She described her baby brother, and, over time, his death. He was crying and her mother screamed, "I'm sick of children!" and got up and shook him. Marianna showed me how her mother shook him, and she showed me what he looked like afterward. A few days later, he died. Marianna was not supposed to see his body in the little casket, but she did. She said they put flowers on his chest. Katya was too little at the time to remember having a baby brother.

The day Peter joined our household as a guest, Dave and I were too busy to pay attention to him. We were having company that night and I was making dinner. Dave mowed the lawn. Katya watched TV with him and they played. Peter made the first move in meeting me. He put Katya's green beanbag cushion on his back and moved around my feet. I though it was Katya. I also thought of the admonition in *Macbeth* to beware of the moving forest. Peter flipped off the cushion and flashed me a megawatt smile. Of course, he knew nothing about *Macbeth*. He was pretending to be a turtle.

Peter blended into our household imperceptibly. He did not fight with the girls or raise his voice. He went to sleep when I put him to bed. The trick to keeping him there was to move him into Marianna's room; that way the two who could not sleep alone had company and everybody got enough rest. He liked the stories I read to him and he was easy to be with.

That summer, *A.I.: Artificial Intelligence* was playing at the movie theaters. When I saw it, I realized Peter was doing the same thing the little robot boy was doing: everything he possibly could to make me love him. He was programmed, just like that robot, to make a mother fall in love with him. I felt guilty because we were not going to adopt him. How could I? I already had two very needy girls. How could I take on a third one and still work full-time?

I put out word that I had a little boy who needed a home. I talked to at least fifty people and got calls from as far away as Atlanta, Georgia. I made arrangements for Peter to meet prospective parents, but it became increasingly difficult for me to tell them how wonderful he was. Peter had succeeded in making me love him. Dave had fallen in love with him three weeks earlier upon bringing him home. Both of us worried that we could not manage three, but we decided we would find a way to do it.

The last week Peter was with us, he had to go to the office with me. I found a Russian-speaking teenager to take care of him during the day so I could work. Fortunately, I work near the National Air and Space Museum, his favorite playground. We fell into an easy routine. We would take Marianna to camp, drive in with my husband, drop him off at work, park the car, and buy lunch on the way to my office. *"Skolka?"* (How many?) I would ask as I pointed to the bananas. The answer was between two and four. Then we would buy two pieces of fried chicken and walk hand in hand to the office. Sometimes we practiced counting in English.

Friday, August 3, was the day he had to return to Russia. We decided to take him by metro to the adoption agency. "Mama, *lubish meenya?*" (Do you love me?) he kept asking. "Yes, Peter," I answered. *"Ya tibya lublyu"* (I love you). I knew in his mind that he wondered, if the answer was yes, why was he going back to Russia? He was frightened when he saw the Russian adoption inspector. She was a wonderful woman, but he knew when he saw her there was no way out. She was escorting the children back home. By chance, he came from the same region in Russia where the girls had lived, and she remembered us from the last time. He clung to me and cried, and even though I had more faith in the system than I had the first time around, my heart broke too. I could not help but think that here was a little boy who came all the way from Russia to find a family, and he succeeded, and now his family was sending him back. I tearfully told another woman who was doing the same thing, "This is the hardest part of the program."

I got my paperwork done faster than anyone else. Part of it had to do with having been down this road before; the rest of it had to do with a sense of commitment. We had made a promise to Peter and we were going to bring him back as soon as possible. This time we were able to call the orphanage from time to time, with Marianna as our main interpreter, so at least he heard our voices, unlike our experience three years earlier when we had no communication with the girls. This time, I found some Russian language cassettes designed for adoptive parents and put more effort into studying them. The alphabet no longer made my eyes cross, though I still haven't learned it, but I can read some things in Russian.

Dave's cousins held a baby shower for us. They gave us all the gifts we needed for the children at the orphanage and the adults with whom we would do business. I supplemented this with a sweep through my closet and included a bottle of cologne I had received for my fortieth birthday but had never opened.

When we had adopted the girls, we had also celebrated our fifth wedding anniversary in Moscow. This time, we flew to Moscow on January 6, 2002, the tenth anniversary of our introduction at a dinner party. When we got there, Eugene, our coordinator from before, greeted us. He took us to the domestic airport for our flight south. This time, we were met by everyone we knew there—Olga, our coordinator; Tina, our translator; and Yuri and Oleg, our drivers. It was a wonderful reunion. They had become like family.

Another American family was on the same flight. They were adopting a little girl from the same orphanage where Peter lived. She was even in his group. They had met their little girl through the Bridge of Hope program too.

The court proceedings went smoothly. The judge remembered us. We visited the girls' orphanage and had lunch with the director and the girls' former caretakers. We gave them photos, visited with the children in their groups, and took more pictures. The orphanage looked like it was better funded. The children were well dressed.

Peter has been with us for only a few months now. His smile lights up my whole being. He's adjusting just fine, making friends, and doing well in school. He actually likes doing homework, and, fortunately, he does not have to overcome the kind of trauma my girls had experienced. He plays games where he sneaks over and kisses my cheek and proclaims, "Gotcha." I always think to myself, "You certainly did." It is wonderful to parent a child who was not abused, but I would not trade my other two for anything. My feisty and sweet little

Katya is rapidly growing up, but she is still my baby chick, her favorite pet name. My beautiful Marianna, the princess, has made remarkable progress. I have heard enough stories about adoptions that did not work out that I do not believe love conquers all, but she certainly has thrived in a nurturing environment that she gets not only at home but also at the wonderful public school she attends.

REFLECTIONS

I know now that adoption is only the beginning of the process, not the end. I am glad we did not know how difficult Marianna was going to be in advance. If we had known, we most likely would not have adopted her, and that thought makes me sad. I am thrilled at the beautiful young woman she is becoming, and a little frightened of what the teenage years might hold. She still has a way to go in coming to terms with her past. She still does not trust anyone completely. I understand why people would not want to take on a child as difficult as she is, but most people I know who have adopted older children have had an easier time. When people tell me that my husband and I have done something few others could do, I disagree. I wish more people would consider it. Finally, I am grateful to the Bridge of Hope program that brought my children to me.

Chapter 13

Four Roads Less Traveled but They All Lead Home

Shirley C. White

My first adoption, at age fifty-nine, was not a calculated, thought-out event, but a culmination of several happenings over a long period of time. I had been employed as a YMCA executive director for several years, then as executive director of a shelter for abused and abandoned children under the age of six years. While my experience with the YMCA was rewarding, the experience with the shelter had a life-changing impact. My adult life had taken place in a middle-class, white culture until I encountered the children and families at the shelter.

FACTORS LEADING TO MY ADOPTIONS

Michelle was my first adoption, in May 1994. She was born in Florida of Haitian parents and was placed in my home in foster care in June 1989 at eighteen months of age. Her health was very fragile and her care very involved. She was an important member of our family, loved by everyone, and she needed the stability and continuity of care I could provide. Michelle was born with AIDS.

Jo was my second adoption. She came to me December 21, 1994, at three months of age, and my adoption of her was the primary goal. She is a very special African-American girl; few adoptive homes

---

The author uses a pseudonym because of confidential information relating to her adopted children, whose need for privacy she wishes to protect. Pseudonyms have been used throughout in order to protect the privacy of those involved and the confidential information disclosed.

would have been available for her because she is HIV positive. Her adoption was finalized November 9, 1995.

Charles's adoption was not planned but came out of love and concern for his entire future if he were to be placed with former relatives, as was planned by the Florida Department of Children and Families (DCF). He too is African American, is hearing impaired, has a history of seizures, and is slightly developmentally delayed, we believe, because of his hearing impairment. He was born HIV positive but has seroconverted. More in-depth information and explanation is given later in the chapter.

A FULL CIRCLE

My life has come full circle. I was placed in an adoptive home at one year of age after my biological mother died of cancer and, a year later, my father hanged himself, leaving six children orphans. Being the baby, I was placed quickly, and my sister, who was a year older, was placed with another family. The oldest girl and three boys were placed in and lived the remainder of their youth in foster care.

My adoptive family was financially poor by most standards but very loving, and they provided me with positive role models, good values, and a strong work ethic. Family was important and big Sunday dinners were the norm. They also had three biological sons. The two older boys accepted me as their little sister, whom they should care for and protect, no matter what. The youngest boy, seven years my senior, was not so protective. He sexually and emotionally abused me and threatened me with "They will send you back where you came from" if I told. Being very young and not knowing I was adopted, I always wondered where I came from. Fear of the unknown and my youth kept me silent. My brother died before I had the opportunity to resolve the abuse issues with him, but through some intense therapy I have learned that he never forgave me for taking his place in the family. I also know now that if I had told my father he probably would have seriously harmed my brother for what he had done, even though my father was a nonviolent man. I was the apple of my father's eye, his pride and joy, but he died several years before my brother did without ever knowing of the abuse. I am at peace with it now, and the happy times in my life are my most vivid and treasured memories. Some of those treasured times are the births of my daughter K. J. and my son Peter and the adoptions of Michelle, Jo, and Charles.

I married young, just eighteen years old, and K. J. was born thirteen months later. I had dated my husband for over three years before we married. He was in the military when we married and had been discharged only three months when K. J. was born. I almost lost her in childbirth, and she was finally delivered by cesarean section. We spent a year paying off the medical expenses for her delivery.

K. J. is now forty-eight years old, has put herself through college, and is working toward her master's degree. She was married, now divorced, and has one son, Scott, who is my pride and joy. Scott graduated from college with honors in May 2001. Both of them have been my strongest supports in the adoptions of Michelle, Jo, and Charles.

My husband and I divorced after six years of marriage and remarried fifteen months later. Peter was born fourteen months after that. Peter is now thirty-nine years old with two health problems, Burger's disease and Raynaud's disease, that threaten his life. He, too, is divorced, with a daughter who will graduate high school this year. He has remarried, and he and his wife are expecting their second child next month. We can only pray on this matter.

My husband and I divorced the second time after another seventeen years of marriage. We parted on amicable terms and remained friends until recently. A rift developed that has created ill will that probably will not be resolved.

While working at the shelter for abused and neglected children, I encountered my first HIV-positive baby, eight-month-old Joey. He was beautiful and had been at the shelter several months prior to my arrival. Once his HIV status was known, the governing board wanted him moved immediately. I tried to explain that the children coming in were more of a threat to him than he was to them. That did not sway them, and Joey was moved. A gentleman came on the board and because of a personal family situation made a contribution to us for research on the need for a special shelter just for HIV-positive babies. A year of work went into the study, obtaining zoning changes and writing grants for the first year of operation. The board was divided. Some thought the stigma would keep other children from being placed in another building on the grounds. Others believed donations would drop significantly. Neither of these dire forecasts proved correct. A few believed in and backed building the shelter. The board and

I could not agree. There were only one or two foster homes for the HIV-positive children, and with the support of a very special person in HRS (Department of Health and Rehabilitative Services), now known as DCF (Department of Children and Families), I left to care for these remarkable children in my own home. I was already licensed as a shelter home.

THE MIRACLE BABY

Michelle, a beautiful little Haitian baby, was placed with me by the Florida HRS in June 1989, at eighteen months of age, with the statement that "she probably will not live thirty days." Michelle had tuberculosis (TB) and had just completed ten days in the hospital being treated for pneumonia and a venereal disease. She had full-blown AIDS and was severely emaciated. She was hospitalized in July 1989 for a few days and again in November 1989 for twenty-seven days. I brought her home in November with instructions to make her comfortable; there was nothing more they could do for her in the hospital that I could not do at home. My prayer was "Please let me have her for Christmas." Then I got greedy and asked, "Can I have her for her birthday?" (which is five days after Christmas). Then I knew we were on borrowed time but it was OK, I said, "I will take whatever You give us." He has given us twelve years and five months, and we are still hopeful.

In the five years Michelle was in foster care with me, she had several social workers, many court appearances, and one adoption worker. Her biological mother died in Haiti and her biological father made a few visits but was unable to care for her. He agreed several times to sign surrender of parental rights forms and then changed his mind. Termination of parental rights was finally initiated by the state. He currently lives in the area and Michelle is free to see him but refuses. He has a daughter one year older than Michelle with him, and she is healthy. Michelle did meet him one time because she had questions she wanted to ask. I have encouraged her to see or contact him again but she does not want to, though maybe someday she will.

Michelle's adoption went smoothly once the father's rights were terminated. My home study for her adoption only had to be updated from my licensing as a foster parent and was completed by Betty, an adoption worker for HRS. While she was supportive, some of my comments about the foster care system and some workers were not well received. In 1994 HIV-positive children were not expected to live more than a few years, so the fact that I am Caucasian and Michelle is Haitian did not become a big concern as it did with my adoption of Charles. Michelle had already lived longer than ever expected.

In 1994 Michelle was accepted for a protocol at the National Institutes of Health (NIH) in Bethesda, Maryland. She was extremely ill and nothing seemed to be working. Her protocol was the three-drug cocktail and it worked. Her CD4 count improved from 149 to over 300 within the year and her viral load dropped from over 200,000 to 20,000 or less. Normal CD4 range is 1,000 to 1,200, and ideally the viral load could be undetectable, meaning less than 500 at that time. In 1994/1995 a viral load of less than 20,000 was a good sign, particularly when it previously had been much higher.

Michelle's care is a daily monitoring responsibility. She has asthma, is prone to severe headaches, has coughing spells that completely wipe her out, is allergic to insect bites, and has frequent nosebleeds.

The unknown or undisclosed factors for these children can be devastating to them as well as to the family in which they are placed. I did not know Michelle's language of origin was Creole until over a year after her placement. I later learned there was a strong possibility of sexual abuse, but the case was never pursued. There was an assumption that she was developmentally delayed because she did not talk. This surely was not true. She just did not understand English. She is shy, reserved, and relatively quiet (except with her close peers) but is not delayed.

On one occasion the foster care worker came to my door, unannounced and unknown to me, bringing with her another foster parent that was to "visit and bond with Michelle so we can move Michelle there." Michelle had been with me three years at that time, her health was very fragile, and she certainly did not need the added stress of moving to an unfamiliar home. Her doctors and I advocated strongly for her not to be moved and were successful. She had been in at least three different placements in the first eighteen months of her life, and my home was her first stable placement and home. She was an integral part of our family by that time and a psychological sibling to the other children in my home, as well as with my biological children. I could not let her go.

Michelle is now a typical fourteen-year-old in many ways. She likes to roller blade, bike, and swim; hang out with her friends; and go to 'NSync concerts. While her energy level can be normal or even high, her stamina is short-lived. She lives because twenty-five pills a day help contain the mutation of the virus, but she also periodically fights and is treated for depression. She has disclosed her HIV status to only two of her friends and lives with the fear that others will find out and their parents won't let them be friends with her. She is living two lives, one secret and one not; this creates an incredible amount of stress that can be devastating to her health. She has a history of cardiomyopathy and was steroid dependent for several years. When she was placed with me, she had TB that had received only sporadic treatment. After a full year of treatment she has been clear for nearly twelve years. She truly is a miracle child, as many of her doctors have called her.

JO ARRIVES ON THE SCENE

Currently Jo is a delightful, enthusiastic, busy, loud, not-to-be-ignored-at-any-cost, seven-year-old, going on twenty-seven, in first grade. She is African American and HIV positive. She is nosy, is eager to be accepted, and is often referred to as "the Camp Director" in our home. She became a permanent member of our family on November 9, 1995. I learned of Jo in late November 1994 through another foster parent. She was in a Children's Home Society foster home in Broward County but they did not plan to keep her because of her HIV status. By now it was well known within the child welfare system that I took in HIV-positive children, aggressively pursued the best treatment for them, loved them with all my heart, without reservations of any kind, and was prepared to see them through to death, if that was to be.

On December 21, 1994, my godson drove me to Broward County to meet and visit with Jo. As much as I wanted to, there was no plan to bring her home. The foster parents were bringing her to the Children's Home Society office for the visit, and her biological mother would be there also. Jo's biological mother wanted to meet the family the society was considering for her placement. I met Jo and the foster parents, who were obviously very attached already. The foster father could hardly stand the thought of losing her, but their family had agreed it was best for Jo and for them for her to be placed in a home more prepared to deal with her health concerns. She clearly had been "Daddy's girl."

The biological mother, Debra, seemed very nice and was well dressed, mannerly, and concerned about where her daughter would go. She had given it a great deal of thought. If Debra became seriously ill and passed on, her mother would have to care for and raise Debra's other three children. She did not believe her mother could stand the stress of losing her, raising the three children, and dealing with Jo's illness. Her decision was to let Jo be adopted. I believe I alleviated any concerns she had. She seemed comfortable with the decision, and I actually got to bring Jo home with me. The understanding was that it was a preadoption placement and something could happen that would interfere with this being finalized. I could bring her home only because I was already a licensed foster home. She came home in a beautiful red and white Christmas suit that I have saved for her.

You can only imagine what Christmas 1994 was like at our house. Two new babies (Jo and Charles), nearly twins; Michelle, five days shy of seven years; Brianna (discussed later), four years; and Santa Claus. It was wonderful, happy, exciting, and thrilling to watch. Their innocence was heart wrenching if you stopped to think about all their other problems. I didn't. We simply lived the day and time to its fullest, as we try to do every day.

The first six months with Jo were not easy. She cried and fussed a lot and was not a happy baby. I had been told she was not drug exposed, but every behavior during that first six months told me differently. When the children were babies we had Nanny Bodi. Bodi had years of experience with children under the best and worst of circumstances. She kept asking in a joking way, "Can we send her back?" By the time Jo was a year old, however, she was a joy to have and busy even at that early age.

Children's Home Society had to complete their own home study on me plus have a letter of support from my biological children, K. J., age forty-one, and Peter, age thirty-two. Children's Home Society visited in my home faithfully each month, but the adoption process went slowly. No particular issue held up the process; it simply had to go through so many different people and receive HRS's consent also.

Jo began her first HIV protocol three months prior to her second birthday at the NIH in Bethesda, Maryland. At the time she was one of the youngest to begin the cocktail antiretroviral treatment for HIV. One of her protocols required us to travel to NIH every other week for thirteen weeks. For over five years her medication schedule was every six hours around the clock: 2 a.m., 8 a.m., 2 p.m., and 8 p.m. I did not deviate from that schedule by more than thirty minutes either way for those five years. It is my firm belief, however, that the early treatment and continuing management of her disease are the primary reasons she remains healthy today. Her viral load is undetectable, meaning less than 200, and her CD4 count is almost within the normal range. She is on medication four times a day now, but it is 6 a.m., 7 a.m., 7:30 p.m., and 8:30 p.m. Her local pediatrician, Dr. C., is nationally recognized in the pediatric HIV field and has been the primary care pediatrician for my children since 1989.

Jo is a snuggler. She likes to be close and needs lots of hugs. She is eager to learn and does well in school. She is also very headstrong and aggressive. She has had to make some adjustments in acknowledging that I am her mother, not her grandmother, and explaining to her friends why she has a white mother. It never was a factor until she went to school, but she has done quite well with all of it. I have been very open with the children about how they came to me and how I have grown to love them. A simple introductory explanation has been that their birth mothers could not take care of them. Jo's friends and their parents have never really questioned the racial difference and. they do not know of her HIV status. I am quite sure Jo may be my biggest challenge yet when she reaches adolescence and her teenage years, but she has been, and continues to be, a delightful addition to our family.

Once again, the unknowns about the children can leave a huge void in many crucial areas. Jo's cholesterol level has been as high as 232 and routinely is over 200. We know one of her medications can contribute to this, but not as significantly as the numbers indicate. We do not know the biological family history in this area. I can pay $100 to pull the records and check what is on file or pay $300 to go back and physically locate the family for that history. I am very concerned about the long-range effects of the high cholesterol in addition to her other health problems.

CHARLES—A FIGHT THAT HAD TO BE WON

Now seven years old, Charles is quite often referred to as my million-dollar man. He is the youngest of my children and became a permanent member of our family only after a three-year legal battle with the Florida Department of Children and Families. Except for the grace of God; Alan M., Esq., my attorney; and Drs. S. and D., the pulmonologist and psychologist involved, we would not have Charles. He, too, is African American.

Charles was eleven days old when I picked him up at the hospital on December 15, 1994. He had been treated for congenital syphilis, tested positive for HIV, and been multiple drug exposed. All the children and Nanny Bodi went with me to get him. Everyone was so excited because it had been quite some time since we had had a baby in the house. He looked like a little old man with a big head and short stubby legs. A very dear friend once described him as "an old soul." I have always said there is no such thing as instant bonding, but there was a special connection with Charles from our first day, and this connection was never broken throughout our three-year battle or since.

During Charles's first six weeks he began having seizures, three within two days, and was put on phenobarbital. His first year was filled with severe otitis (ear infections), and by the time he was eighteen months old he was diagnosed with asthma. He also had seroconverted, meaning he no longer was HIV positive. He had shed his birth mother's antibodies for the virus. He was healthy! Tubes were put in his ears to help with the otitis.

The day Charles's ear tubes were placed was remarkable. He ran his fingernail down textured wallpaper and heard the sound for the first time. After we got home and the doorbell rang he nearly jumped out of my arms. He obviously had not heard it before. I laughed for joy that he could hear and cried for his pain and lost opportunities because of his hearing loss. When I went into the nursery, many times Charles did not appear to know I was there until a loud noise or vibration reached him. Jo could be bouncing in her crib and Charles would not hear her. A test of his hearing showed the loss was moderate in one ear and moderate to severe in the other ear. His hearing fluctuates and we do not know if it will get worse. We do know it will not get better, and his particular hearing loss does not qualify for the cochlear implant. He now wears two hearing aids. His new "ears," as he calls his hearing aids, will be digital and programmable.

Parental rights were terminated when Charles was fourteen months old, and he was legally available for adoption at fifteen months of age. The birth mother had thirty days in which to appeal the termination, but she did not appeal. A former relative who had two of Charles's half siblings then came forward and stated that she wanted Charles as a foster child, but not to adopt. She had known about him since birth but had made no attempt prior to this to gain custody. I had agreed to "bridge" Charles by the book to his new home *if* DCF found him an *appropriate permanent placement*. He was not to linger in foster care because of his disabilities or because he had been HIV exposed and had seroconverted. I knew of children who had been introduced to prospective adoptive parents and then been rejected because of their HIV exposure, even though they had seroconverted. If any of these things happened, then Charles was to be mine.

I met the relative after the termination trial and gave her a big picture of Charles. She seemed nice and appeared to be sincere. Visits at McDonald's began and continued for about six or seven months. Charles liked going to McDonald's to play. Then overnight visits started. Charles cried every time he was removed from our home and put into a car with either the DCF worker or the relative. The DCF worker insisted I put him in his car seat so he would understand I was giving him permission to go. I finally refused to carry him to the car crying, kicking, holding on to me, and screaming "No, no, no!" It was very clear he did not want to go. On the first visit after he got his first hearing aid he rolled the window down and threw his hearing aid away. The relative did not know he had done so because he was in a car seat behind her. She had taken Charles to a pediatrician in her town to have him checked because she did not believe he needed his seizure and asthma medications. While they were there she discovered his hearing aid was missing. She remembered that he had rolled the window down and threw what she had thought was a toy out the window. Most of the times he visited in her home he was not given his seizure medication or nebulizer treatments for his asthma. I measured and documented his medications before and after every visit. On all visits except one, he was either given the incorrect dosage or not given medicine at all. By now he was visiting every other weekend. This continued for several months.

Throughout this time of visitation in the relative's home, Charles came home with his clothing and even his hair smelling of smoke. I would immediately wash all of his clothing or place it in an airtight bag until it was washed, then put him in the bathtub and wash his hair. When I discussed this with DCF, they said they would let the relatives know that Charles could not be around smoke while he was in their home. Still he continued to come home with the smoke odor. An emergency court order finally stopped the overnight visits. I later learned that both parents in the home smoked.

Charles started preschool the day after his third birthday, talking very little, being extremely shy and undoubtedly unsure of himself. He did not know where he belonged. When the overnight visits stopped, his teachers could not believe the change in him and the exceptional progress he began to make. Their quote was, "He blossomed!"

When the relatives first asked to take Charles, they wanted him in long-term foster care. This would have allowed the birth mother access to him at any time. The board payment for foster care was considerably larger than the subsidy that would go with his adoption—approximately $450 versus $275. DCF had, without my knowledge, gone back to court and had Charles's permanency goal changed from adoption to long-term foster care. I learned about it quite by accident three months after the fact. Long-term foster care was, and is, against the law since parental rights had been terminated and an adoptive home was available; thus, adoption was mandated. I had filed to adopt by that time.

I spoke with my attorney, Alan M., about the actions of DCF in reversing Charles's legal status from adoption to long-term foster care. He said it was not legal and they could not do that. He agreed to write them a letter. In less than three weeks Charles's permanency goal was changed back to adoption. By this time we also had his negative HIV tests, and knowing this the relatives then decided they would adopt Charles. This was not an appropriate placement for Charles. They vacillated between adoption and foster care for months, finally agreeing to adopt. While the mother in that family was four years younger than I, the father was ten years older. The half siblings, who were in long-term foster care and living with these relatives, were ten and eleven years older than Charles and able to care for themselves. There were four other half siblings scattered throughout south Florida. The biological mother did not have custody of any of them.

The legal fight for Charles's best interests began in August 1996 and ended July 12, 1999. Not one person in the child welfare system disagreed with HRS. The guardian ad litem, Foster Care Citizens Review, and Human Rights Advocacy Committee all recommended Charles be removed from my home and placed with his relatives. One group even stated he should be removed from my home and placed in another foster home if he could not be placed with the relatives immediately. Their reasoning was that I was too attached to Charles. The Human Rights Advocacy Committee agreed that Charles's civil right to permanency within the time frame defined by the law had been violated but still recommended he be moved. While many children in care do not have a guardian ad litem because there are not enough, Charles had two. DCF had its own attorney on the case, then late in the case hired two outside attorneys.

All of the various agencies and departments considered biological half sibling connections as the major factor in removing Charles from our home. Those connections simply did not exist. During a deposition the psychologist who evaluated Charles addressed the fact that his psychological siblings were the children in my home, not his biological half siblings. I certainly believe this was one of the most important turning points in the case. Three of Charles's biological half siblings he had never even met, and there were no plans in place for him to meet them.

On at least two occasions DCF attempted to move Charles with twenty-four hours or less notice. I was preparing for Michelle's birthday party on December 30, 1998, when I received the call to have Charles in HRS's office between 10:00 a.m. and 11:00 a.m. the next morning. He was being moved to the relatives. DCF knew the judge on the case was out of town for the holidays. Alan M., my attorney, and I went to the Fourth District Court of Appeals in West Palm Beach the next morning to ask for an emergency hearing and stay until the regular judge on the case returned. Our request was granted just minutes before Charles was to be moved. It surely dampened the festivity of Michelle's birthday and the family's New Year's celebrations. It is difficult to revisit the memory even now.

We made one trip north for my grandson's graduation. I had permission to take Charles out of state. We left a day and a half earlier than planned because my sister had been found in a diabetic coma. This was the second time in less than three weeks. Later when I checked my messages I learned DCF had wanted to keep Charles in Florida and put him in the relatives' home while we were gone. If that had happened it would have been very difficult, if not impossible, to get him back. I am sure Charles would never have understood and would have felt lost and abandoned had he been left behind. All the children were excited about going because they would see K. J. and Peter and it had been so long since we had been out of town.

I was accused of controlling the doctors providing care for Charles. It was alleged that I exhibited symptoms of Munchausen by proxy in "causing" his illnesses. There were times that I felt hopeless, discouraged, and alone. I moved from being used as a shining example of a great foster parent and advocate for the children in my home, respected within the system, to being exiled by that same system. I had taught foster-parenting classes for DCF for seven or eight years, two or three of those years without compensation, but I believed so strongly in the program and how it could help the children that I paid a baby-sitter and continued to teach anyway. I have not been asked to teach one class since filing for the adoption of Charles. Without the strong support of my daughter, K. J., close friends, Alan M., and Charles's specialty doctors, I could not have endured. I went from despair to elation or elation to despair. Only a few very close friends, my attorney, and K. J. saw those highs and lows. While my son Peter could not physically be present, he gave lots of verbal support. Court dates were a regular occurrence. K. J. flew in twice from out of state for support during court appearances. Everything at home had to continue as near normal as possible. Medications had to be given and doctor's appointments kept. Trips to NIH were crucial. Vacations were forfeited because of the lack of money and because we did not dare leave town for fear of what might happen while we were gone. Life stood still but did not stand still.

The unknowns about Charles remain just that. I have little biological medical history on him. He has asthma, a history of seizures, is hearing impaired, and wears two hearing aids. He has two biological half siblings who are hearing impaired, so I do not know if it is caused by an inherited trait, exposure to HIV and syphilis, or a combination of all of these. In the final adoption I agreed for him to see and visit with the relatives. It was a precedent-setting adoption visitation agreement giving him the best of both worlds. The relatives have not contacted me since the finalization of the adoption.

On July 14, 1999, an editorial in the *Palm Beach Post* newspaper, "Finally, [Charles] Goes Home," told the story in brief form:

> that she [Ms. White] had to file a civil rights lawsuit to do so is a travesty. . . . Perhaps DCF resisted because [Ms. White] has criticized the agency. The settlement includes a pledge by DCF not to retaliate against her. . . . Arrogance and intransigence cost the public $135,000, to pay [Ms. White's] legal bills, and nearly cost a 4-year-old boy a loving home.

Lawsuits to Protect Children's Rights

Four lawsuits were pending at one time during my effort to adopt Charles. The first was for my adoption of Charles, then one on behalf of Michelle and Jo for discrimination under the Americans with Disabilities Act. The third one was filed for civil rights violations, and the last against One Church/One Child.

A reference to children in the home being "terminally ill" was one of the reasons for not placing Charles in our family. This was a direct reference to the HIV status of Michelle and Jo and, under the Americans with Disabilities Act, an expressed discrimination against them.

The focus of the civil rights suit against the Florida DCF was based on some of the same factors: the girls' HIV status, an indirect reference to my age, and a statement that Charles belongs with his own "culture," an oblique reference to race. Charles is black and I am white. Nearly every point on which DCF based their recommendations against allowing me to adopt him was discriminatory.

One Church/One Child is a program, legislated and funded by the state of Florida through the One Church One Child Corporation Act, that asserts every black child belongs in a black home. Again, it is discriminatory and illegal. That lawsuit was settled in civil court for $1.00. The program still exists even though its mission is discriminatory and its major funding source is the state of Florida.

My attorney fought every motion filed from every approach possible. Nearly all of the time he had, in advance, thought the possibilities through so thoroughly that our motions were filed first. It was a struggle, sometimes even a battle, to gain access to the information DCF had. All of the suits were transferred to one juvenile court, Judge

Ronald A. presiding, with the exception of the One Church/One Child suit.

Charles's cases were followed closely by child welfare personnel, child advocates, foster parents, and attorneys. They received national coverage. Several people wrote editorials and called radio talk shows. The results of the adoption finalization were picked up by the Associated Press. There was overwhelming support from outside our county and state.

BRIANNA—A VERY DIFFERENT STORY

I have full custody, from the state of Florida, of twelve-year-old Brianna, who has complex mental health difficulties. She arrived in our home in July 1990 at nine weeks of age, after a three-week hospitalization for malnutrition that had led to cardiac arrest. She has been diagnosed as bipolar with paranoid schizophrenic indicators; with oppositional defiant syndrome, attention-deficit hyperactivity disorder (ADHD), and reactive attachment disorder (RAD); and is HIV positive. Brianna's first signs of emotional difficulties became evident as early as three years of age. Her attachments were out of need, not out of love. She was completely self-absorbed and showed no signs of remorse for hurting other children. The only teacher who could control her behaviors in preschool was a man. When he was not in the classroom, Brianna destroyed property and totally disrupted the classroom. When she was five years old, parental rights were terminated and I asked for guardianship rather than to adopt. There were several reasons to take that course of action. First, mental health services for children are practically nonexistent in our geographic area, and, secondly, I had no idea how serious Brianna's difficulties were or would become. I also had to consider my age and that if anything happened to me, my daughter K. J. would assume full responsibility for all of the children. She needed options to be open to her depending on Brianna's mental health, and with consideration being given to all of the children's physical health. Brianna is a 24/7 responsibility and may have to be placed in a residential treatment program sometime in the future. She can and does severely limit the family's activities at times. I have learned not to take her to any important events where her behavior could disrupt the event or embarrass the other children. It is impossible to know or even guess what will set her off on a screaming, kicking, running, hitting tirade. It can be anything from a simple request for a pencil to her having to admit to stealing—my cell phone, her brother's Game Boy, forty dollars from her sister, or anything else she sees that she wants. Certain activities and places are to be avoided. She attends a class for severely emotionally handicapped (SEH) children in school, which has been very good for her. Her physical health is satisfactory and has remained stable for several years.

Brianna's biological history is sketchy. Her father is unknown and her mother has a history of violence, drug abuse, and prostitution. She is the third generation of her family to be on welfare, with family arrests dating back two generations on various drug-related charges. Her future is most uncertain. I have often said, "I can't get old; Brianna won't let me."

A RETROSPECTIVE GLANCE

I have learned so much with each adoption. With Michelle the most difficult part was keeping her stabilized and in my home while she was still in foster care. Since she was not expected to live very long, age and race did not impede the adoption process, which actually progressed very quickly once her father's rights were terminated. Jo's finalization took nearly a year through Children's Home Society. I'm not sure why because her mother had signed the requisite surrender papers. The three-year legal fight to adopt Charles took its toll on the entire family, especially him. However, during that three years he was, on many occasions, the stabilizing factor amid the chaos. His personality and humor were the glue that held us together.

Charles's case reiterates, over and over, the need for high-quality adoptive homes that can provide a stable, loving, secure, permanent environment for each and every child available for adoption, regardless of mitigating factors. Foster care is, hypothetically, short-term, temporary care. Unfortunately, that is not what happens in most cases. Far too many children spend years or even their entire childhood in foster care. That should not be an option. Discrimination based on race, age, gender, or any other reason should not stand in the way of permanency for any child. Discrimination for any of those reasons, as well as others, is illegal.

The costs for adoption through the state are normally underwritten by the state. Some small up-front costs are reimbursed, but that process can be very slow. I could have picked from a list of attorneys provided by DCF, with legal fees related to adopting paid directly to that attorney, or chosen another attorney, paid him or her myself, and waited for reimbursement by the state. In the latter case, the total amount was preset and if the attorney's fee was more, the extra cost was mine. This is not true in an adoption that is contested in any way, such as Charles's. All costs relating to Charles's adoption were mine. DCF had to reimburse my direct expenses because we won. If we had lost, the entire bill would have been mine.

The past fourteen years have been the most satisfying of my life, in addition to the years I spent raising K. J. and Peter. I believe I am finally doing what I was meant to do. Once these inimitable children have touched your life, you are never the same. I have learned what really is important in life, how to be spontaneous and to seize and make the most we can of every day and, in some cases, of every moment. The ups and downs of the children's health are like a rollercoaster ride. You ride to the heights and pray a lot when you are at the bottom. I refuse to look too far down the road. My parents told me that worry is interest on a loan that 95 percent of the time is never taken out. In the down times I try hard to remember that. If I have one regret, it would be that I did not adopt Theodore, a foster child I had once and lost to death.

Chapter 14

Problems, Perils, and Pleasures of Mulitcultural and Biracial Adoptions

Florence W. Kaslow

As one reads the preceding chapters, several themes and trends become apparent. These will be extrapolated and highlighted in this final chapter, but, first, a few preliminary comments on the raison d'être for this book and the methodology used in selecting contributing authors.

In our travels throughout the United States and many other countries, it has become abundantly clear that more and more adults are adopting children from countries other than the one in which they reside. The question "Why is this occurring?" tantalized us. We decided, since the majority of the books on adoption have been written by those who work professionally in some aspect of the adoption field, that a book written primarily by those who had personally done the adopting, the parents, would add a unique perspective. We hypothesized that the most kaleidoscopic portrait could be rendered by having multiple authors, rather than just one or two, and that we should seek parents with diverse backgrounds in terms of education, occupation, geographic locale, socioeconomic strata, and marital status.

However, the method of selection was definitely not random. We began by inviting people we knew, friends and acquaintances, to participate and received a very favorable response. As we told more people about this adventure on which we were embarking, they recommended others, and these were added to the list of potential contributors. We tried to include parents who had adopted from a variety of countries and succeeded to some extent. However, most, but not all, cluster around China, Russia, and Romania—possibly because it was well publicized that that these countries had many children available for adoption in the 1980s and 1990s. Yet some of our other authors adopted from Cambodia, Greece, Iran, Latvia, Poland, and Thailand, so the range is fairly diverse and broad. We tried repeatedly to find someone who had adopted from Central or Latin America but never quite finalized any connection. For example, one Chilean psychiatrist who agreed to submit a chapter never followed through, despite repeated reminders. Nonetheless, we are extremely pleased that two of our authors reside in Sweden, thus allowing us to offer a broader perspective emanating from two different cultural contexts.

Because we used a network sampling method (Kuzel, 1992), we started with people we knew and they then referred their acquaintances; thus, the vast majority of the authors (or their spouses) fall within the professional category of occupations. They are predominantly lawyers, psychologists and psychiatrists, journalists, etc. It is possible that this also reflects the reality that the preponderance of people who engage in multicultural/international adoptions are college educated, upper middle to upper class economically, and employed in high-level professional and business occupations. It is hypothesized that since these adoptions are costly, require enormous patience and perseverance, and depend on the ability to navigate the legal and immigration systems of two countries, people with fewer financial resources and a less cosmopolitan worldview might be less apt to contemplate, much less undertake, such a long-term journey.

The group of parents who are the contributing authors are mostly heterosexual married couples. In this category, two of the chapters are authored by the fathers. Our sample also includes one lesbian couple and two single mothers. Hopefully this contributes to a more multidimensional view of the kinds of adults who have a desire to be parents and offer good parenting to children whose birth parents are unable and/or unwilling to raise them. In these personal narratives, poignantly written from the heart as well as the mind, one hears and can almost visualize all the drawn-out deliberations that went into the decision to adopt and then to embark on the circuitous international adoption pathway. All describe the numerous interviews entailing very personal questions and home studies, usually with social workers, to see if they "qualify" and if their homes are suitable (an experience common in domestic adoptions as well). Once approved, the long and costly journeys abroad begin, and sometimes they return home without the promised child. They recount the arduous process of working with lawyers here and/or abroad, as well as with intermediaries, or "facilitators" as they are often called, who may or may not be trustworthy; flying overseas and then traveling hundreds of miles over strange terrain to get to the orphanage or the pickup site; staying in uncomfortable hotels that do not meet their usual and customary standards; having to pass Bureau of Citizenship and Immigration Services (formerly INS) requirements and procedures in two countries; and finding that the baby or child they receive often is developmentally delayed and may have numerous physical and medical problems.

REASONS FOR SEEKING TO ADOPT ABROAD

Nonetheless, all but one of the authors chose to adopt a child from another country for such reasons as the following:

1. There were many more foreign-born than U.S.-born babies and older children available.
2. They were/are altruistically and humanistically motivated to provide loving parenting to a child (children) who might otherwise be destined to spend his/her (their) childhood and adolescent years in an orphanage.
3. Some of the requirements for becoming adoptive parents have been less restrictive in such countries as Russia, Poland, and China than in the United States or Sweden.
4. Several who are quite religious felt they had received a strong message from G_D that they should adopt a foreign-born child, in one instance from a particular country, Romania—when its overcrowded and substandard orphanages were very much in the news.
5. They had a definite preference for a closed adoption so that they would not have to worry that the child's (children's) biological parent(s) would resurface to claim the child (children) they had grown to love or that they would encounter other future legal complications.

MULTICULTURAL ISSUES

Chapter 13 by Shirley C. White is unique in this collection in that the children she adopted are American-born, hard-to-place children—several of whom were HIV positive, and several of whom are African American while she is Caucasian. Her chapter poses the interesting dilemma that social agencies in the United States, such as Children's Aid Societies, will place special needs children with parents of a different race for foster care, but if and when adoption becomes possible, many people, such as African-American ministers and social workers, make a strong case for African-American children to be placed only in an African-American family. (The same argument has been made by some Native American tribal leaders; thus, the stance is not unique to only one specific racial or ethnic group.) White cogently argues for a different stance, that is, children should be placed in the best home available for them at the time of the placement, and that race and ethnicity constitute one salient factor but that there are many others, most notably continuity of loving care and not severing attachment bonds that have been forged. We see in her chapter and in the writings of the numerous parent-authors who adopted Asian children, who are also visibly different from their Caucasian parents, that their "love is color blind," and that bonding and caring for a child who is different encompasses a much more transcendent ability to become attached because of a heart connection.

It does not appear that any of these parents engage in denial about the differences in racial background or country of origin. Rather, they fully accept and value the differences. For example, several of the parents with daughters from China (Moro, Chapter 4; Allen, Chapter 5; Morris and Jones, Chapter 6) arrange for their daughters to maintain close contact with other Chinese children adopted by Caucasian parents, on a personal level and through organizations set up specifically for this purpose. The children celebrate the Chinese New Year, as well as other holidays that reflect and typify their heritage, often with their Chinese peers. Parents who have adopted children from Romania and Russia also meet so that their children can share common roots and they can interact with other parents as a mutual support group (Berman, Chapter 10). The meetings may be picnics or other types of gatherings that occur one or more times a year. Lieberman and Bufferd (1998) offer a number of suggestions for family acknowledgement of the special meaning of adoption in the book *Creating Ceremonies*. Some of the parents have taken their children back to visit the homeland of their birth (Moessinger, Chapter 3; Cederblad, Chapter 8), recognizing the importance of their children's knowing about their roots, being proud of them, and incorporating all of these facets of their being into their total sense of identity. Many of the parents have kept scrapbooks and photo albums documenting their adoption journeys, the orphanage and the caretakers there, the celebrations "welcoming home" the children to their new lives here, and daily and major events in the children's and families' lives subsequent to the adoptions. The bicultural and multicultural kinds of families that these families personify have become more numerous in the past decade and are less often objects of curiosity. Furthermore, these parents believe that the two (or more) parts of a family's identity make it more interesting and stimulating, as well as more challenging.

Several intimate indirectly or indicate directly that the long, circuitous, cumbersome adoption process, including the filling out of myriad papers and the multitudinous meetings and miles traveled, can be considered comparable to and a metaphor for the usual period of pregnancy—only longer. The costs involved are quite variable for both, the range being greater with adoption unless fees have some set cap, as with the Swedish agency regulated by government-approved fees. Fee schedules are obviously something that each potential adoptive parent needs to check out as fully as possible before embarking on this pathway, and we recommend trying to have these put in writing, with all possible contingencies noted, so they are legally binding. We realize this may not always be possible.

As indicated earlier, when they arrive, many of the children evince developmental delays. These range from mild to serious, depending on numerous factors, including how old they are when adopted, how much stimulation they did or did not receive in the orphanage in which they resided, their own genetic makeup, etc. However, all report that their children caught up quickly once they felt secure and received a great deal of love, attention, and stimulation. Many spurt ahead of the norm and become high achievers (see, for example, Palmer, Chapter 11).

COPING WITH UNCERTAINTIES
AND NEW REALITIES

At some level, all the adults had been aware that the child they received may well have had some physical problems (Allen, Chapter 5; Cederblad, Chapter 8; Kaufman, Chapter 9), and they were all willing to undertake coping with this, providing their physicians believed the condition to be correctible (Allen, Chapter 5; Kaufman, Chapter 9). Less known were the emotional problems that the child might already have internalized—particularly if the child had been exposed to neglect, abuse, and other severe trauma and was more than a year and half old at the time of the adoption. Perhaps the most extreme example of this is contained in Anne's chapter (Chapter 12), in which she discusses her three Russian-born children, the trials and tribulations in acquiring them, and the turbulence that had been pervasive in her two daughters' lives while with their biological mother in Russia. Yet all persevered during the tumultuous times, seeking therapy for themselves and their children when needed, and hoping and praying that love, guidance, stability, and predictability ultimately would lead to the child developing into a sound, well-integrated, healthy person.

Palmer (Chapter 11) relates that adopting a daughter from Romania into his blended family, which already had three children, worked out so well over time that they responded to her request for her older sister to join their family, and his wife went back to Romania to bring her home too.

Two chapters have addenda from "grown children." Chapter 3 by Moessinger contains an addendum by her daughter, Deborah, who was adopted several decades ago. She recapitulates what the experience has meant to her, thus providing a fuller picture from two different perspectives. Dunne (Chapter 7), who decided to adopt when her several biological children were grown, graciously invited these four children and her mother to write their comments in separate addenda. They take us through their feelings of astonishment, uncertainty, curiosity, and joy regarding their mother/daughter's adoption of two foreign-born children who became an integral and dearly beloved part of their family. These kaleidoscopic, multigenerational portraits provide a unique contribution to the extant literature.

One common expectation is that the child might be the object of teasing outside of the family orbit because he or she looks different from the parents, although this is less common today in many communities than it would have been twenty or thirty years ago. They all attempt to help their children be prepared to cope with this by providing possible answers and explaining why the teasing occurs.

REFLECTIONS

It is not possible to mention each chapter separately, but this synopsis of the portraits of the parent-authors is intended to be inclusive. All appear to be open-minded, liberal, flexible, courageous, tenacious, willing to take risks, and altruistic. They hold realistic expectations for their children, understanding they will not get "perfect children." All have a deep desire to have one or more children. They agree that the children should be exposed to their cultural and ethnic roots and explain as much about their heritage as possible in an age-appropriate manner, with perhaps those portions which would be too denigrating of their biological parents omitted.

They manifest great honesty and integrity as they tell their stories, including discussions of their misgivings and, in some instances, the slowness with which the deeper level of bonding occurred and the acting out or shyness diminished. Many of the parents indicate they later contributed to supporting the orphanages from which they acquired their children, hoping to help them stay afloat to take care of the many needy children entrusted to them and to continue their efforts in placing these children in the arms of those who want them, sometimes desperately. Almost all allude to having taken gifts of toys, clothing, and money to the orphanages (directly or through intermediaries) when they went to claim their children.

We gave the contributing authors a choice between writing under their own names or under pseudonyms. Both options were selected. Several decided that they wanted to protect their identities and those of their children, not wanting to open their private lives to scrutiny or any possible risk. Most wrote under their real names, and some willingly and proudly submitted photographs. We posit that this represents a fair microcosm of possible reactions to the idea of public disclosure, particularly to a large and unknown audience, such as anonymous readers of a book or magazine.

Some make sound suggestions for potential adoptive parents, such as obtain videos and pictures of the child, take these to a physician who specializes in international adoptions for whatever medical clearance can be ascertained from these, and on arrival home quickly take the child to a pediatrician to have a baseline evaluation done and any existing conditions treated. They also suggest buying open airline tickets since one cannot be sure that the return home will take place according to the anticipated schedule, explaining that sometimes the circumstances can be discussed with the airlines and exceptions to the usual rules and regulations will be made. In addition, prospective parents should familiarize themselves with the rules governing international adoption in their home country and in the country from which they are adopting—and be aware that these change frequently—so they stay abreast of these changes. Sometimes there are advisories on the Internet about State Department concerns that prospective parents can check.

Despite all of the exigencies entailed, most of the parents decided to adopt a second, third, or even fourth child. What better testament could there be to the tremendous value they place on their children and the indisputable fact that the positives far outweigh the difficulties and the negatives?

LEGAL CONCERNS

The State Department has received a growing number of complaints concerning adoption facilitators operating in various countries. Licensing of agents and facilitators is done in accordance with local laws. Unfortunately, not all foreign governments require that agents and facilitators be licensed. Accordingly, it can be difficult to hold facilitators accountable for fraud, malfeasance, or other bad practices in general. Under these circumstances, the State Department cannot endorse individual adoption facilitators in a given country.

We strongly urge citizens contemplating international adoption to retain the services of a reputable adoption agency licensed by one or more of the states in the United States, or by their own country, if not the United States, and also to work with a reputable attorney who specializes in immigration law. The attorney should also be familiar with adoption law. Adopting parents should question their agency about the qualifications and experience of any facilitators it might use in a foreign country and the degree to which the agency assumes responsibility for the actions of its agents or facilitators. We encourage adopting parents to consider carefully their decision to use a particular agency if that agency asserts that it is not responsible for the actions of its agents or facilitators.

Adopting parents should check with the state licensing agencies and consumer protection agencies, such as the Better Business Bureau, regarding the qualifications of and possible complaints against adoption agencies. Contact information for state licensing agencies is available from the National Adoption Information Clearinghouse (NAIC) at <http://www.calib.com/naic/database/nadd/naddsearch.cfm>. Adopting parents may also check with the various national organizations of adoption agencies. Information regarding these organizations also is available on the NAIC Web site at <http://www. calib.com/ naic/database/nat/schorgs.cfm>.

There are numerous Web sites on the Internet that adopting parents can check for information, including complaints, regarding adoption service providers. Please note, however, that the State Department cannot endorse nor assume any responsibility for the content of these Web sites (see the appendix for adoption resources).

A recent article in the *New York Times Magazine* (Corbett, 2002) cautions that "American parents adopting Cambodian children have reason to wonder if the babies were bought or coerced from their mothers. There are legitimate adoptions, but since a corrupt system erases a baby's past, few parents can know for sure." It is a chilling account of some of the underhanded practices allegedly found in connection with some Cambodian adoptions and adds some balance to the otherwise predominantly rosy picture that has emerged from our parent-authors.

POSTSCRIPT

We have attempted to ground this overall tapestry in the current research in the field as reported by Lipton and colleagues (Chapter 2). Actually, their findings, based on a large sample in which they studied 1,489 adopted children and their families (the Northeast-Northwest Collaborative Adoption Project), run quite parallel to what our authors, individually and collectively, recount—particularly how much the children have enhanced their lives and how glad they are that they were able to make such journeys to welcome their children home.

We hope this book will help others decide if international, multicultural, and/or biracial adoptions are for them and, if so, serve as a guidebook to help chart their course of action and offer encouragement when they hit the inevitable bumps along the road.

REFERENCES

Corbett, S. (2002). Where do babies come from? *New York Times Magazine,* June 16, pp. 42-47, 74, 82-83.

Kuzel, A. J. (1992). Sampling in qualitative inquiry. In B. F. Crabtree and W. L. Miller (Eds.), *Doing qualitative research* (pp. 31-44). Newbury Park, CA: Sage.

Lieberman, C. A. and Bufferd, R. K. (1998). *Creating ceremonies: Innovative ways to meet adoption challenges.* Phoenix, AZ: Zeig, Tucker, and Theisen, Inc.

Appendix

Adoption Resources

IN THE UNITED STATES

American Academy of Adoption Attorneys
P.O. Box 33053
Washington, DC 20033

Children's Hope International Adoption Agency
<http://childrenshopeint.org>

Evan B. Donaldson Adoption Institute
6 East 94th Street
New York, NY 10128

Families for Russian and Ukranian Adoption (FRUA)
<http://www.frua.org>

Joint Council on International Children's Services
(adoption agency should be a member of this)
<www.jcics.org>

National Adoption Information Clearinghouse
11426 Rockville Pike, Suite 410
Rockville, MD 20852

National Council for Adoption
225 North Washington Street
Alexandria, VA 22314-2520
(703) 299-6633

PACT, An Adoption Alliance
Becca Martinson
3450 Sacramento Street, #239
San Francisco, CA 94118

Rainbow Kids
(online source of information on international adoption)
<www.rainbowkids.com>

Resolve
(organization concerned with infertility and its alternatives)
1310 Broadway
Somerville, MA 02144

Spence-Chapin Services
6 East 94th Street
New York, NY 10128
(212) 369-0300

U.S. State Department—Office of Children's Issues
(information on international adoption)
<http://travel.state.gov/children's_issues.html>

Welcome House Social Services of Pearl S. Buck Foundation
P.O. Box 181, Green Hills Farm
Perkasie, PA 18944
(215) 249-1516
<www.pearlsbuck.org>

Publications

Adoption Quarterly
The Haworth Press, Inc.
10 Alice Street
Binghamton, NY 13904

Adoption Report
Child Welfare League of America
CN 94
300 Raritan Center Parkway
Edison, NJ 08818

Adoptive Families
Perspectives Press, Inc.
P.O. Box 90318
Indianapolis, IN 46290-0318

OUTSIDE THE UNITED STATES

Canada

Adoption Horizons
Diane Lametti, Catholic Adoption Group
c/o Catholic Adoption Centre
26 Maitland Street
Toronto, Ontario M4Y 1C6

Adoption Roundup
Adoption Council of Ontario
3216 Yonge Street, 2nd Floor
Toronto, Ontario M4N 2L2

Adoptive Parents Association of Nova Scotia (newsletter)
Box 2511, Stn. M
Halifax, Nova Scotia B3J 3N5

Focus on Adoption, Adoptive Parents Association of British Columbia
Suite 205, 15463-104th Avenue
Surrey, British Columbia V3R 1N9

Society of Special Needs Adoptive Parents (SNAP) (newsletter)
409 Granville Street, Suite 1150
Vancouver, British Columbia V6C 1T2

Sweden

Forbundet Adoptionscentrum
Box 1520
S-172 29 Sundbyberg
Smidesvagen 1 Sweden
Phone: 0046-8-587 499 00

Publications

International Adoption Bulletin
Adoption Centre
University of Utrecht, Heidelberglaan 1
3584 CS Utrecht, The Netherlands

Bibliography

Alexander, R., Jr., and Curtis, C. M. (1996). A review of empirical research involving the transracial adoption of African American children. *Journal of Black Psychology, 22,* 223-235.

Babb, L. A. (1999). *Ethics in American adoption.* Westport, CT: Bergin and Garvey.

Berger, D. (1995). Improving the safety and efficiency of foreign adoptions: U. S. domestic adoption programs and adoption programs in other countries provide lessons for INS reform. *Cornell Journal of Law and Public Policy, 5,* 33-65.

Cohen, N. J., Coyne, J., and Duvall, J. (1993). Adopted and biological children in the clinic: Family, parental and child characteristics. *Journal of Child Psychology and Psychiatry, 34,* 545-562.

Connelly, L. M. (1993). Adoption of Carlos: Blood thicker than law in Massachusetts. *New England Law Review, 28,* 515-542.

Daly, K. (1988). Reshaped parenthood identity: The transition to adoptive parenthood. *Journal of Contemporary Ethnography, 17,* 40-66.

Groothues, C. L. M., Beckett, C. M., and O'Connor, T. G. (2001). Successful outcomes: A follow-up study of children adopted from Romania into the UK. *Adoption Quarterly, 5*(1), 5-22.

Hollingsworth, L. D. (1998). Promoting same-race adoption for children of color. *Social Work, 43,* 104-116.

Isaacs, A. D. (1995). Interracial adoption: Permanent placement and racial identity—An adoptee's perspective. *National Black Law Journal, 14,* 126-156.

Koch, R. L. (1992). Transracial adoption in light of the foster care crisis: A horse of a different color. *New York Law Journal of Human Rights, 10,* 147-184.

Lieberman, C. A. and Bufferd, R. K. (1998). *Creating ceremonies: Innovative ways to meet adoption challenges.* Phoenix, AZ: Zeig, Tucker and Theisen, Co.

Liow, S. J. R. (1994). Transracial adoption: Questions on heritage for parents, children and counsellors. *Counseling Psychology Quarterly, 7,* 375-384.

Lippold, J. M. (1995). Transnational adoption from an American perspective: The need for universal uniformity. *Case Western Reserve Journal of International Law, 27,* 465-503.

Mainemer, H., Gilman, L. C., and Ames, E. W. (1998). Parenting stress in families adopting children from Romanian orphanages. *Journal of Family Issues, 19,* 164-180.

Mannis, V. S. (2000). The adopting single mother: Four portraits of American women adopting from China. *Adoption Quarterly, 4*(2), 29-55.

McRoy, R. G. (1997). Achieving same-race adoptive placements for African American children: Culturally sensitive practice approaches. *Child Welfare, 76,* 85-104.

Murphy-Berman, V. and Weisz, V. (1996). U.N. Convention on the Rights of the Child. *American Psychologist, 51,* 1231-1233.

Newman, L. E. (1992). Jewish theology and bioethics. *The Journal of Medicine and Philosophy, 17,* 309-327.

Pertman, A. (2000). *Adoption nation: How the adoption revolution is transforming America.* New York: Basic Books.

Rosnati, R. and Marta, E. R. (1997). Parent-child relationships as a protective factor in preventing adolescents' psychosocial risk in inter-racial adoptive and non-adoptive families. *Journal of Adolescence, 20,* 617-631.

Schooler, J. E. and Norris, B. L. (2002). *Journeys after adoption: Understanding lifelong issues.* Westport, CT: Bergin and Garvey.

Shanley, M. L. (2001). *Making babies, making families.* Boston: Beacon Press.

Shapiro, V. B., Shapiro, J. R., and Paret, I. H. (2000). *Complex adoption and assisted technology.* New York: Guilford Press.

Steinberg, G. and Hall, B. (2000). *Inside transracial adoption.* Indianapolis, IN: Perspectives Press.

Vacek, E. C. (1992). Catholic "natural law" and reproductive ethics. *The Journal of Medicine and Philosophy, 17,* 329-346.

Varon, L. (2000). *Adopting on your own: The complete guide to adopting as a single parent.* New York: Farrar, Straus, and Giroux.

Verhulst, F. C., Althaus, M., and Versluis-den Bieman, H. J. M. (1990). Problem behavior in international adoptees: II. Age at placement. *Journal of the American Academy of Child and Adolescent Psychiatry, 29,* 104-111.

Wardle, F. (1990). Endorsing children's differences: Meeting the needs of adopted minority children. *Young Children, 45,* 44-46.

Wasser, S. K., Sewall, G., and Soules, M. R. (1993). Psychosocial stress as a cause of infertility. *Fertility and Sterility, 59,* 685-689.

Wetzstein, C. (1998). Adoption advocates encouraged by big response to internet sites. *Insight on the News, 14*(4), 40-41.

Zisk, M. (2001). *The best single mom in the world: How I was adopted* [for children]. Morton Grove, IL: Albert Whitman and Co.

Index

Page numbers followed by the letter "i" indicate illustrations.